UROLOGIC ROBOTIC SURGERY

CURRENT CLINICAL UROLOGY

Eric A. Klein, SERIES EDITOR

Urologic Robotic Surgery, edited by **Jeffrey A. Stock, Michael P. Esposito, and Vincent J. Lanteri,** 2008

Genitourinary Pain and Inflammation: Diagnosis and Management, edited by **Jeanette M. Potts,** 2008

Prostate Biopsy: Indications, Techniques, and Complications, edited by **J. Stephen Jones,** 2008

Female Urology: A Practical Clinical Guide, edited by **Howard Goldman and Sandip P. Vasavada,** 2007

Urinary Stone Disease: The Practical Guide to Medical and Surgical Management, edited by **Marshall L. Stoller and Maxwell V. Meng,** 2007

Peyronie's Disease: A Guide to Clinical Management, edited by **Laurence A. Levine,** 2006

Male Sexual Function: A Guide to Clinical Management, Second Edition, edited by **John J. Mulcahy,** 2006

Advanced Endourology: The Complete Clinical Guide, edited by **Stephen Y. Nakada and Margaret S. Pearle,** 2005

Oral Pharmacotherapy of Male Sexual Dysfunction: A Guide to Clinical Management, edited by **Gregory A. Broderick,** 2005

Urological Emergencies: A Practical Guide, edited by **Hunter Wessells and Jack W. McAninch,** 2005

Management of Prostate Cancer, Second Edition, edited by **Eric A. Klein,** 2004

Essential Urology: A Guide to Clinical Practice, edited by **Jeannette M. Potts,** 2004

Management of Benign Prostatic Hypertrophy, edited by **Kevin T. McVary,** 2004

Pediatric Urology, edited by **John P. Gearhart,** 2003

Laparoscopic Urologic Oncology, edited by **Jeffrey A. Cadeddu,** 2004

Essential Urologic Laparoscopy: The Complete Clinical Guide, edited by **Stephen Y. Nakada,** 2003

Urologic Prostheses: The Complete Practical Guide to Devices, Their Implantation, and Patient Follow-Up, edited by **Culley C. Carson, III,** 2002

Male Sexual Function: A Guide to Clinical Management, edited by **John J. Mulcahy,** 2001

Prostate Cancer Screening, edited by **Ian M. Thompson, Martin I. Resnick, and Eric A. Klein,** 2001

Bladder Cancer: Current Diagnosis and Treatment, edited by **Michael J. Droller,** 2001

Urologic Robotic Surgery

Edited by

Jeffrey A. Stock, MD

*Children's Hospital of New Jersey,
Newark, NJ and Mount Sinai School of Medicine,
New York, NY*

Michael P. Esposito, MD

*Center for Minimally Invasive Urologic Surgery,
Hackensack University Medical Center,
Hackensack, NJ*

Vincent J. Lanteri, MD

*Center for Minimally Invasive Urologic Surgery,
Hackensack University Medical Center,
Hackensack, NJ*

Foreword by

David M. Albala, MD

*Department of Urology,
Duke University,
Durham, North Carolina*

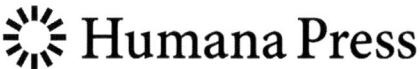 Humana Press

Editors
Jeffrey A. Stock
Children's Hospital of New Jersey
Newark, NJ and
Mount Sinai School of Medicine
New York, NY
USA
Jeffrey.Stock@mountsinai.org

Michael P. Esposito
Center for Minimally Invasive Urologic Surgery
Hackensack University Medical Center
Hackensack, NJ
USA
mikevino@aol.com

Vincent J. Lanteri
Center for Minimally Invasive
   Urologic Surgery
Hackensack University Medical Center
Hackensack, NJ
USA

Series Editor
Eric Klein, MD
Professor of Surgery
Cleveland Clinic Lerner College
   of Medicine
Head, Section of Urologic Oncology
Glickman Urological and
   Kidney Institute
Cleveland, OH

ISBN: 978-1-58829-615-3   e-ISBN: 978-1-59745-128-4

Library of Congress Control Number: 2007940758

Cover illustration: Intuitive Surgical, Sunnyvale, CA.

Printed on acid-free paper

9 8 7 6 5 4 3 2 1

springer.com

This book is dedicated to our wives Esther, Jennifer, Susan, and to our children, Ari, Yosef, Dina and Michael, Abrianna and Marissa, Alexis, Elizabeth.

Foreword

The introduction of robotic technology into modern day operating theatres has changed the way that surgery will be performed. The last 5 years have shown a paradigm shift toward the adoption of robotic surgical techniques by private and academic institutions alike. For example, in just 4 years, the number of radical robotic prostatectomies alone has increased from a mere 300 to over 16,000 in 2005. This transition has been driven by an increasingly educated patient population who seek out less morbid ways to address their disease. The introduction of this new technology has allowed for a significant advancement in patient care. By providing a minimally invasive surgical option, patient recovery is faster with outcomes comparable to open surgical techniques.

Despite the increasing popularity of this technology, there remains a dearth of literature available to surgeons and patients. Drs. Jeffrey Stock, Michael Esposito, and Vincent Lanteri are to be commended for providing one of the most useful textbooks on robotics in urologic surgery. This textbook has been organized to be as complete as possible in presenting accepted robotic applications to treat common urological problems.

The book begins with a chapter on the history of robotic surgery. Following this, a description of basic instrumentation and techniques is presented. Chapters follow on specific techniques that are structured to discuss potential applications as well as contraindications. As each procedure is described, attention is given to patient positioning and trocar placement. Detailed directions given in the text demonstrate the critical steps for each procedure. The last section of the book reviews robotic suturing, complications, and training and credentialing.

For the practicing urologist, this text serves as a needed educational guide to understanding the scope of robotic procedures performed. This book is written in a way that clinicians, researchers, and in parts lay people will understand and appreciate. It is a comprehensive book that will be an invaluable addition to every urologist's library.

David M. Albala, MD
Duke University,
Durham, North Carolina

Contents

Foreword vii
Contributors.. xiii

PART I: HISTORICAL PERSPECTIVE

1   History of Robotic Surgery   3
    Ilya A. Volfson and Jeffrey A. Stock

PART II: SETUP AND ACCESS

2   Operating Room Setup, Patient and Instrument
        Preparation...   29
    Laura Wisse

3   Port Placement and Exit   39
    Rahuldev S. Bhalla

PART III: ROBOTIC LAPAROSCOPIC PROCEDURES

4   Robotic Transperitoneal Four Arm Laparoscopic Radical
        Prostatectomy: Points of Technique   49
    Sagar R. Shah and Vipul R. Patel

5   Extraperitoneal Robotic Radical Prostatectomy   71
    Michael P. Esposito, Vincent J. Lanteri, and Gregory Lovallo

6   Robotic Laparoscopic Radical Cystectomy   89
    Jay Yew and Timothy Wilson

7   Robotic Laparoscopic Nephrectomy, Partial Nephrectomy,
        and Nephroureterectomy 111
    Jay Yew

8   Robotic Donor Nephrectomy................................. 125
    *María Verónica Gorodner, Carlos Galvani, Enrico Benedetti,
    and Santiago Horgan*

9   Robotic Pyeloplasty 139
    Jeffrey A. Stock, Michael P. Esposito, and Gregory Lovallo

10 Robotic Ureteral Reflux Surgery 145
    Joseph G. Borer and Craig A. Peters

11 Robotic Orchiopexy... 159
      Bartley G. Cilento and David Diamond

PART IV: OTHER CONSIDERATIONS FOR ROBOTIC SURGERY

12 Robotic Suturing... 171
      Scott J. Belsley and Garth H. Ballantyne

13 Hemostasis.. 185
      Ayal M. Kaynan

14 Complications of Robotic Surgery........................... 199
      Joseph R. Wagner and Caner Z. Dinlenc

15 Policy Guidelines for Robot-Assisted Surgery in Urology 207
      *Ralph Madeb, Joy Knopf, Gregory Oleyourryk,
      Louis Eichel, and John R. Valvo*

16 Anesthetic Considerations for Laparoscopic Procedures
      in Urology... 215
      *Leslie M. Leaf, Daniel C. Leaf, Robert S. Dorian,
      and Mark Hausdorff*

Index 229

DVD Contents

4   Robotic Transperitoneal Four Arm Laparoscopic Radical
        Prostatectomy: Points of Technique
        Sagar R. Shah and Vipul R. Patel

5   Extraperitoneal Robotic Radical Prostatectomy
        Michael P. Esposito, Vincent J. Lanteri, and Gregory Lovallo

6   Robotic Laparoscopic Radical Cystectomy
        Jay Yew and Timothy Wilson

7   Robotic Laparoscopic Nephrectomy, Partial Nephrectomy,
        and Nephroureterectomy
        Jay Yew

8   Robotic Donor Nephrectomy
        *María Verónica Gorodner, Carlos Galvani, Enrico Benedetti,
        and Santiago Horgan*

9   Robotic Pyeloplasty
        Jeffrey A. Stock, Michael P. Esposito, and Gregory Lovallo

10 Robotic Ureteral Reflux Surgery
        Joseph G. Borer and Craig A. Peters

11 Robotic Orchiopexy
        Bartley G. Cilento and David Diamond

12 Robotic Suturing
        Scott J. Belsley and Garth H. Ballantyne

Contributors

GARTH H. BALLENYTNE, MD • *Director, Section of Minimally Invasive and Telerobotic Surgery, Hackensack University Medical Center, Hackensack, NJ*

SCOTT J. BELSLEY, MD • *Fellow, Section of Minimally Invasive and Telerobotic Surgery, Hackensack University Medical Center, Hackensack, NJ*

ENRICO BENEDETTI, MD • *Department of Surgery, University of Illinois, Chicago, IL*

RAHULDEV S. BHALLA, MD • *Director of Minimally Invasive Surgery, Division of Urology, New Jersey Medical School, Newark, NJ*

JOSEPH G. BORER, MD • *Department of Urology, Children's Hospital Boston, Boston, MA*

BARTLEY G. CILENTO, MD • *Department of Urology, Children's Hospital Boston, Boston, MA*

DAVID DIAMOND, MD • *Department of Urology, Children's Hospital Boston, Boston, MA*

CANER Z. DINLENC, MD • *Director, Division of Endourology and Stone Disease, Department of Urology, Beth Israel Medical Center, New York, NY*

ROBERT S. DORIAN, MD • *Chairman, Department of Anesthesiology, Saint Barnabas Medical Center, Livingston, NJ*

LOUIS EICHEL, MD • *Division of Urology, Rochester General Hospital, Rochester, NJ*

MICHAEL P. ESPOSITO, MD • *Co-Director, Center for Minimally Invasive Urologic Surgery, Department of Urology, Hackensack University Medical Center, Hackensack, NJ*

CARLOS GALVANI, MD • *Department of Surgery, University of Illinois, Chicago, IL*

MARÍA VERÓNICA GORODNER, MD • *Department of Surgery, University of Illinois, Chicago, IL*

MARK HAUSDORFF, MD • *Director, Section of Pediatric Anesthesiology, Children's Hospital of New Jersey, Newark, NJ*

SANTIAGO HORGAN, MD • *Director Minimally Invasive Surgery, Department of Surgery, University of Illinois, Chicago, IL*

AYAL M. KAYNAN, MD • *Section of Urology, Department of Surgery, Morristown Memorial Hospital, Morristown, NJ*

JOY KNOPF, MD • *Division of Urology, Rochester General Hospital, Rochester, NJ*

VINCENT J. LANTERI, MD • *Center for Minimally Invasive Urologic Surgery, Department of Urology, Hackensack University Medical Center, Hackensack, NJ*

DANIEL C. LEAF, MD • *Resident, Department of Anesthesiology, Saint Barnabas Medical Center, Livingston, NJ*

LESLIE M. LEAF, MD • *Resident, Department of Anesthesiology, Saint Joseph's Medical Center, Patterson, NJ*

GREGORY LOVALLO, MD • *Center for Minimally Invasive Urologic Surgery Department of Urology, Hackensack University Medical Center, Hackensack, NJ*

RALPH MADEB, MD • *Division of Urology, Rochester General Hospital, Rochester, NJ*

GREGORY OLEYOURRYK, MD • *Division of Urology, Rochester General Hospital, Rochester, NJ*

VIPUL R. PATEL, MD • *Director, Center for Robotic Surgery, Department of Urology, The Ohio State University, Columbus, OH*

CRAIG A. PETERS, MD • *Chairman, Department of Urology, University of Virginia, Charlottesville, VA*

SAGAR R. SHAH, MD • *Department of Urology, The Ohio State University, Columbus, OH*

JEFFREY A. STOCK, MD • *Director, Section of Pediatric Urology, Children's Hospital of New Jersey, Newark, NJ; Chief, Pediatric Urology, Mount Sinai School of Medicine, New York, NY*

JOHN R. VALVO, MD • *Division of Urology, Rochester General Hospital, Rochester, NJ*

ILYA A. VOLFSON, MD • *Chief Resident, Section of Urology, Department of Surgery, University of Medicine and Dentistry, New Jersey Medical School, Newark, NJ*

JOSEPH R. WAGNER, MD • *Department of Urology, Hartford Hospital, Hartford, CT*

TIMOTHY WILSON, MD • *Director, Department of Urology and Urologic Oncology, City of Hope National Medical Center, Duarte, CA*

LAURA WISSE, RN, CNOR • *Clinical Coordinator Laparoscopic and Robotic Surgery, Hackensack University Medical Center, Hackensack, NJ*

JAY YEW, MD • *Department of Robotics & Minimally-Invasive Urologic Surgery, Sharp Memorial Hospital, San Diego, CA*

I Historical Perspective

1 History of Robotic Surgery

Ilya A. Volfson and Jeffrey A. Stock

If every instrument could accomplish its own work, obeying or antic-
ipating the will of others ...If the shuttle could weave, and the pick
touch the lyre, without a hand to guide them, chief workmen would not
need servants, nor masters slaves.

—ARISTOTLE

Robotics, although still an intriguing and exotic concept, much less remote from the life of an average American household than one tends to believe. In the past 70 years, humanoid robots that were supposed to be made with man's physique in mind have captured the public's imagination through numerous science fiction novels and cinematography. Keeping these truly rare creatures aside, we are getting more and more accustomed to various items of our work environment and households that come under the definition of a robot. So, what is a robot?

Using Webster's Dictionary, a robot is as follows: **1 a :** a machine that looks like a human being and performs various complex acts (as walking or talking) of a human being; *also* **:** a similar but fictional machine whose lack of capacity for human emotions is often emphasized **b :** an efficient insensitive person who functions automatically **2 :** a device that automatically performs complicated often repetitive tasks **3 :** a mechanism guided by automatic controls. **Synonyms:** android, automaton

And using the same Webster's Dictionary, robotics is a technology dealing with the design, construction, and operation of robots in automation.

The vision of a nonhuman form performing man's task is far from novel. It can be traced throughout the folklore of most of the cultures from Nordic tribes of Scandinavia to the nomadic tribes of Arabia. One can recall the "self-propelling" boots, flying carpet, magical cook pots, flying

From: *Current Clinical Urology: Urologic Robotic Surgery*
Edited by: J. A. Stock, M. P. Esposito, and V. J. Lanteri © Humana Press, Totowa, NJ

brooms and, off course, the ultimate "non-human slave"—an all-mighty Genie of "Thousand and one nights."

The first automaton creation is credited to a Greek inventor, Ctesibius of Alexandria, in 250 B.C. He developed *clepsydra*, a water clock that substituted a cumbersome sand clock. Sand clock was designed as such that a keeper had to turn it upside down every time an upper chamber ran out of sand. Clepsydra, on the other hand, did not require a man-keeper and therefore is considered to be the first automaton in human history.

As humans evolved in their craftsmanship and scientific knowledge, their aspirations grew. Their imagination turned toward the unthinkable— creation of the mechanical replica of self. Our knowledge of the first humanoid automaton dates to the Renaissance era. Leonardo da Vinci, the ultimate "Renaissance man," a great artist, engineer, and scientist is credited with the first design of a humanoid automaton. It is still unknown whether an actual model was ever built, but several design drawings have been discovered in the 1950s among the lost da Vinci's writings (Figs. 1–5).

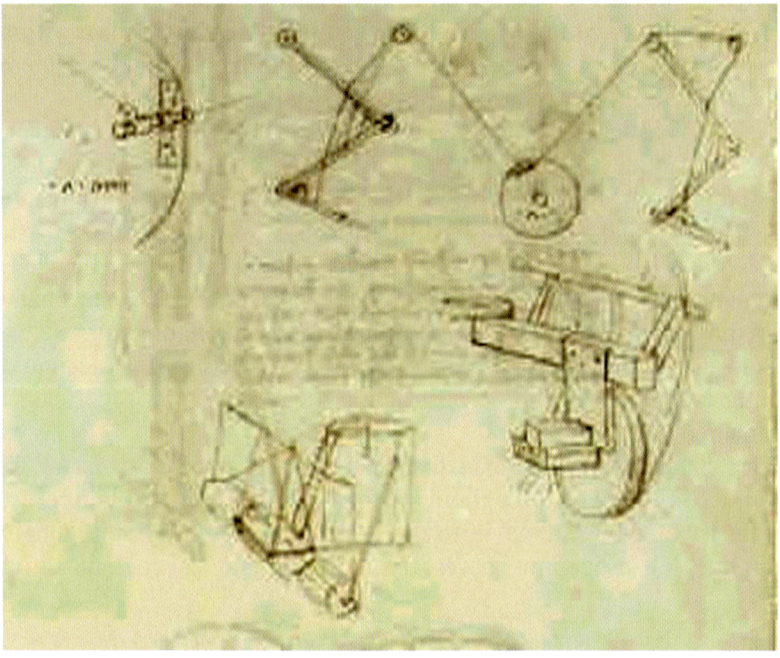

Fig. 1. Design drawings of the lost da Vinci writings (from Institute & Museum of the History of Science, Florence, Italy).

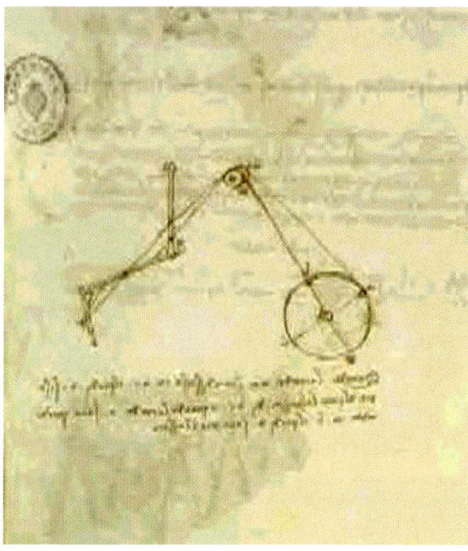

Fig. 2. Design drawings of the lost da Vinci writings (from Institute & Museum of the History of Science, Florence, Italy).

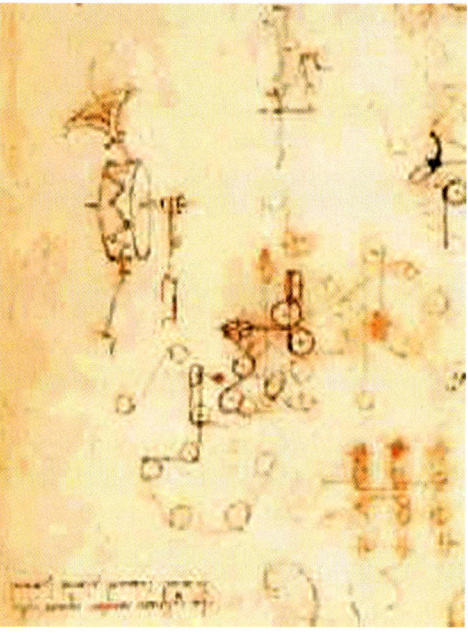

Fig. 3. Design drawings of the lost da Vinci writings (from Institute & Museum of the History of Science, Florence, Italy).

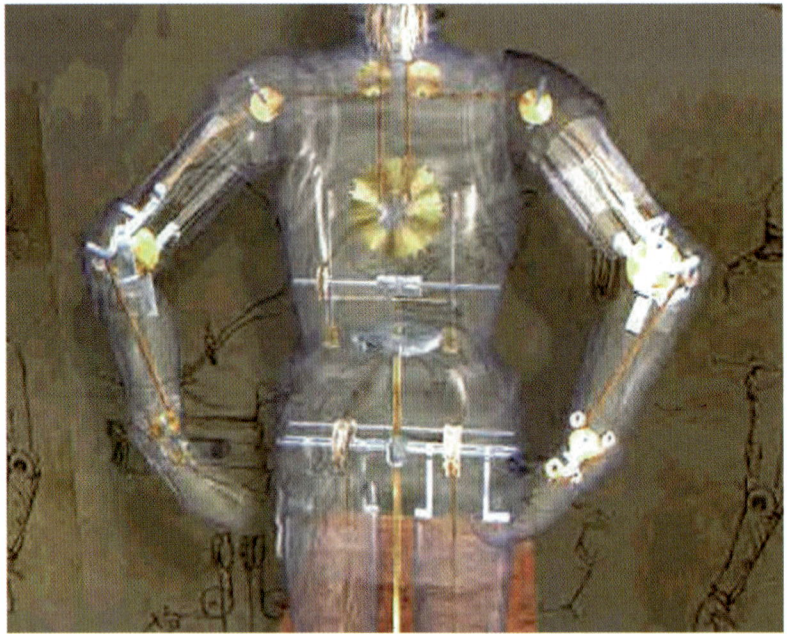

Fig. 4. Design drawings of the lost da Vinci writings (from Institute & Museum of the History of Science, Florence, Italy).

After scrupulous processing with computer models developed by Florence-based Institute and Museum of the History of Science, newly found drawings were determined to be the design sketches for a model of a medieval knight. The drawings date to 1495, shortly prior to Leonardo's "last supper period." The knight was designed according to the Vitruvian cannon. One can marvel at Leonardo's knowledge of anatomy, recorded in the Codex Huygens, and the armored robot knight was a direct extention of that knowledge. The robot was designed to sit up, wave its arms, and move its head via a flexible neck, while opening and closing its anatomically correct jaw. It may have made sounds to the accompaniment of automated drums. Off note, the famous invention was recently popularized in the bestselling novel "The da Vinci Code" by Dan Brown.

The record of the first mechanical automaton that started appearing throughout Europe dates to the eighteenth century. The world's first successfully build automaton is the famous *Flute Player* (Fig. 6), constructed by the French engineer Jacques de Vaucanson in 1737 (Fig. 7). And his most famous creation was the mechanical duck that was built in 1741 (Fig. 8). It could flap its wings, eat, and digest grain. Each wing contained >400 moving parts, and even today the complexity of

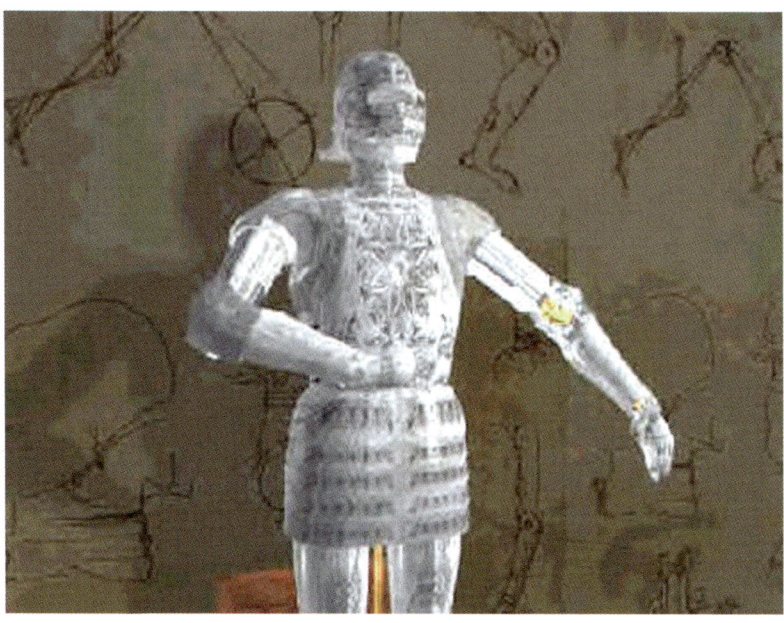

Fig. 5. Design drawings of the lost da Vinci writings (from Institute & Museum of the History of Science, Florence, Italy).

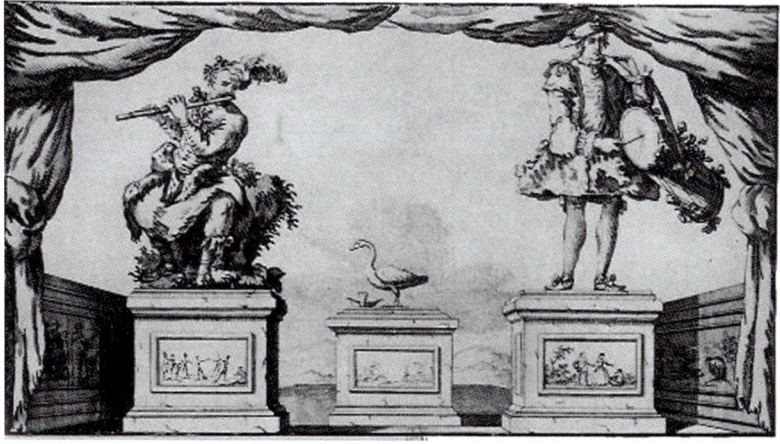

Fig. 6. Automaton Flute Player by Jacques de Vaucanson (from http://www. tecsoc.org/pubs/history/2002/nov21.htm).

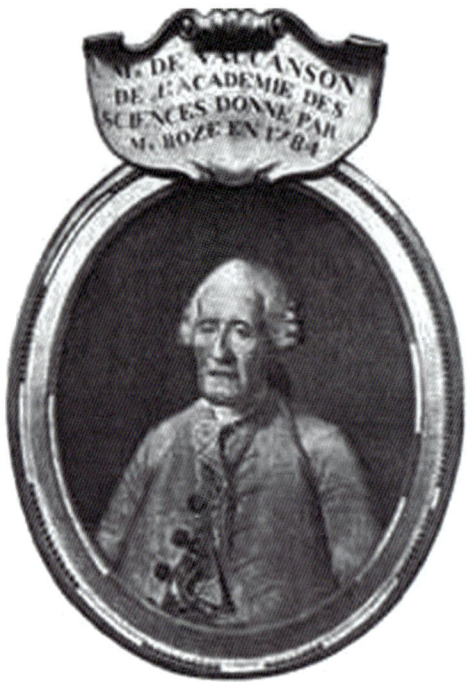

Fig. 7. Jacques de Vaucanson (from http://www.tecsoc.org/pubs/history/2002/nov21.htm).

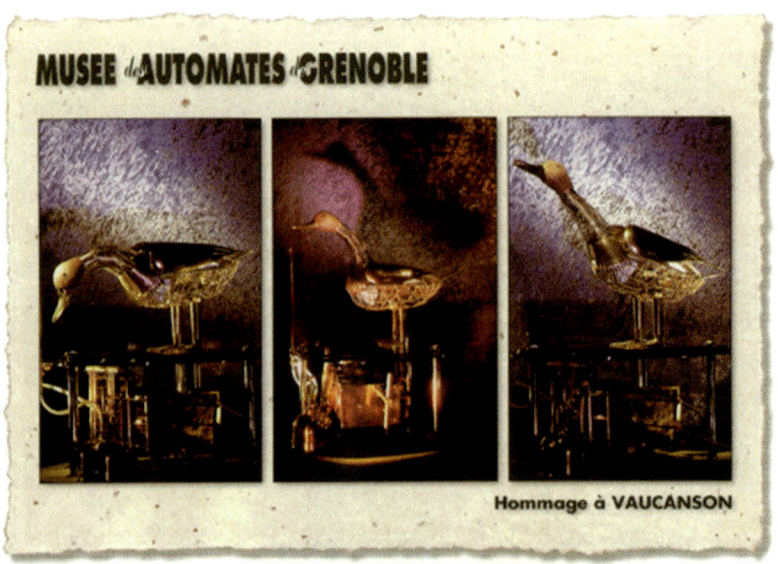

Fig. 8. The automaton duck by Jacques de Vaucanson (from http://www.tecsoc.org/pubs/history/2002/nov21.htm).

design remains somewhat of a mystery. Unfortunately, the original duck has not survived to present. Voltaire once wrote about de Vaucanson: "A rival to Prometheus, [Vaucanson] seemed to steal the heavenly fires in his search to give life."

Another famous automaton was created by the Swiss mechanician Henri Maillardet, which was capable of drawing four pictures and writing three poems. Restored to its original capabilities the automaton is now part of the collection at The Franklin Institute Science museum in Philadelphia (Figs. 9–11).

The world first remote-controlled vehicle was build by Croatian-American scientist Nikola Tesla (Fig. 12). At the time when understanding of radio waves was primitive at best, he introduced his radiocontrolled submarine at the scientific fair in New York City at the turn of 20th century. The invention was so much ahead of its time that many in the

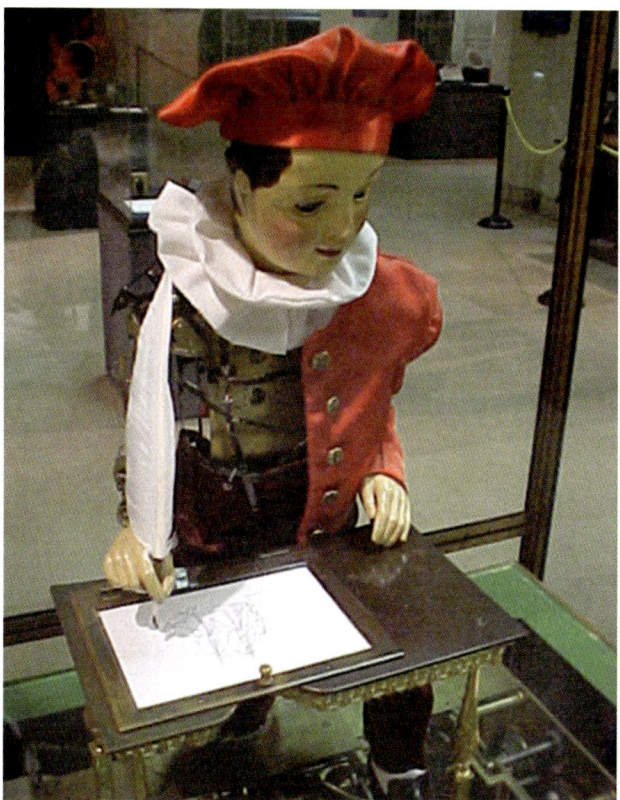

Fig. 9. Automaton by Henri Maillardet (from Franklin Institute, Philadelphia, PA; http://fi.edu/pieces/knox/automaton/).

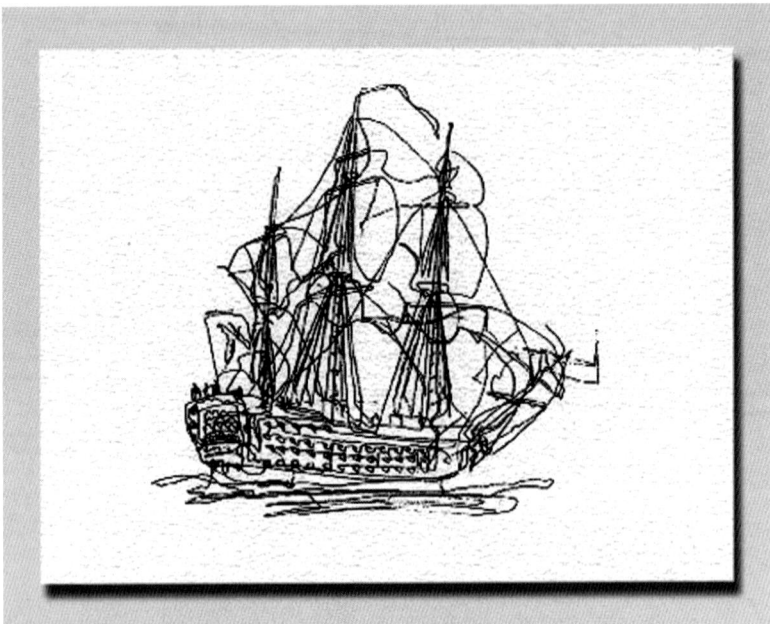

Fig. 10. Ship drawing done by the Henri Maillardet automaton (from Franklin Institute, Philadelphia, PA; http://fi.edu/pieces/knox/automaton/).

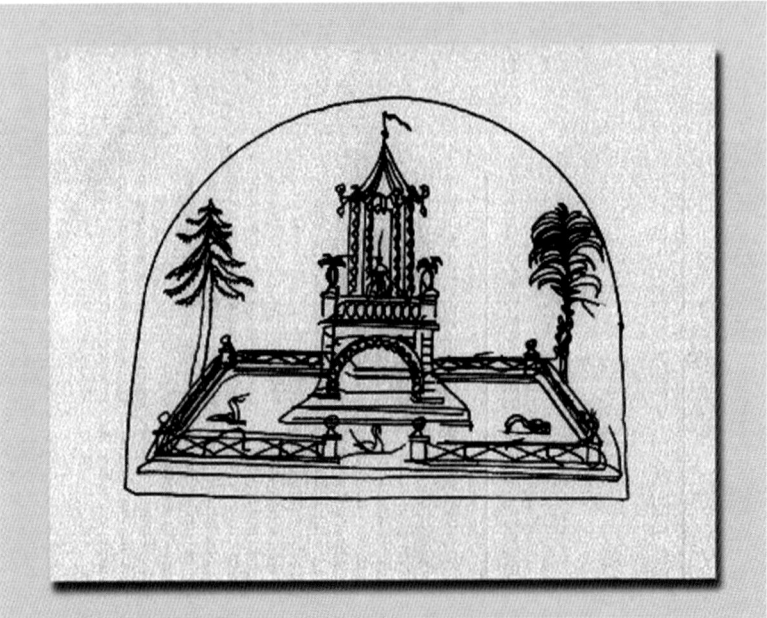

Fig. 11. Chinese structure drawing done by the Henri Maillardet automaton (from Franklin Institute, Philadelphia, PA; http://fi.edu/pieces/knox/automaton/).

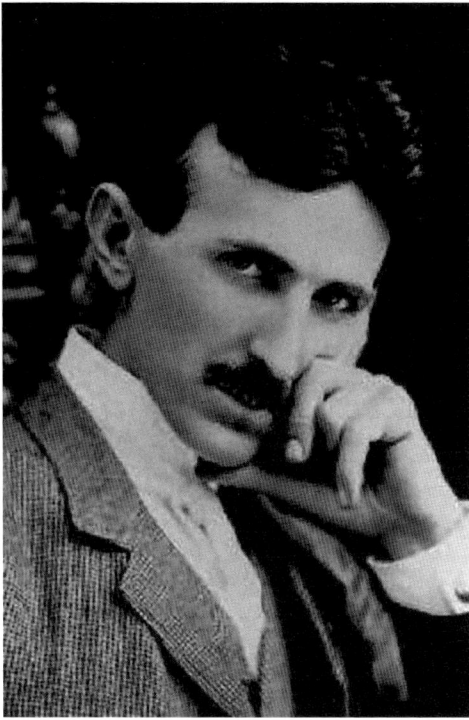

Fig. 12. Portrait of Nikola Tesla (from www.classictesla.com).

audience were convinced that a midget was placed into the machine to operate it under water.

The term "robot" was coined by Karel Capek, Czech play writer, in his 1921 play "R.U.R." (Rossum's Universal Robots) (Figs. 13 and 14). The term was given to electronic servants that, once given emotions, turned against the humans. The term comes from the Czech word "robota," which means "forced labor." The term "robotics" first appeared in Isaac Asimov's "Runaround" (1942) that was later included in his famous book "I, Robot" (Fig. 15).

The involvement of the robots in the 20th century became widespread and versatile. No history of robots and robotics would be complete without mentioning of Asimov's 3 laws of robotics:

1. A robot may not injure a human being, or, through inaction, allow a human being to come to harm.
2. A robot must obey the orders given it by human beings except where such orders would conflict with the First Law.
3. A robot must protect its own existence as long as such protection does not conflict with the First or Second Law.

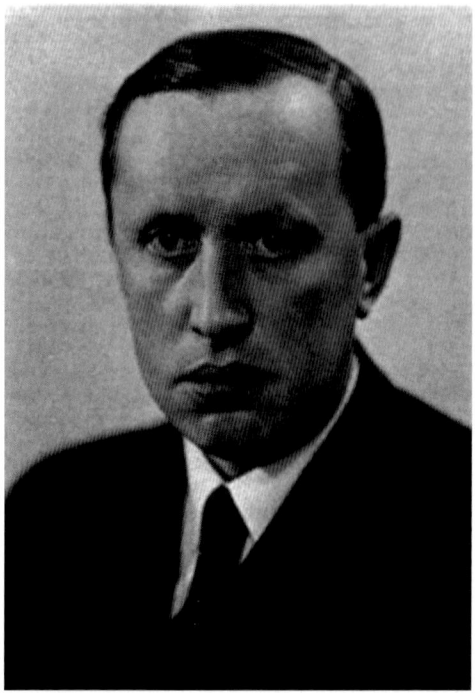

Fig. 13. Portrait of Karel Capek (from http://capek.misto.cz/obrazky/portrety/portraits.html).

The role of the robot became not only to simplify human existence but also to protect its master by taking upon itself various dangerous tasks. The U.S. military developed an automatic system for mine detection that would sit in front of the tank, and, once a mine was detected, it would stop the tank before it got too close to the mine. Obviously, law enforcement readily invested in this new field. Robots are widely implemented now in testing suspicious packages in airports and in deactivation and detonation of explosive devices. Robotics found its application in various fields during and after World War II. With modern warfare turning toward the domination over the sky, radar (another form of a robot) became essential in tracking the enemy. Military continued with its heavy investment in robotics with drone planes and armored vehicles that are now part of the U.S. military.

Industry quickly recognized an enormous potential for robots. In 1961, General Motors installed its first robotic system to the assembly line. In 1978, Programmable Universal Machine for Assembly (PUMA) was first introduced and quickly gained popularity.

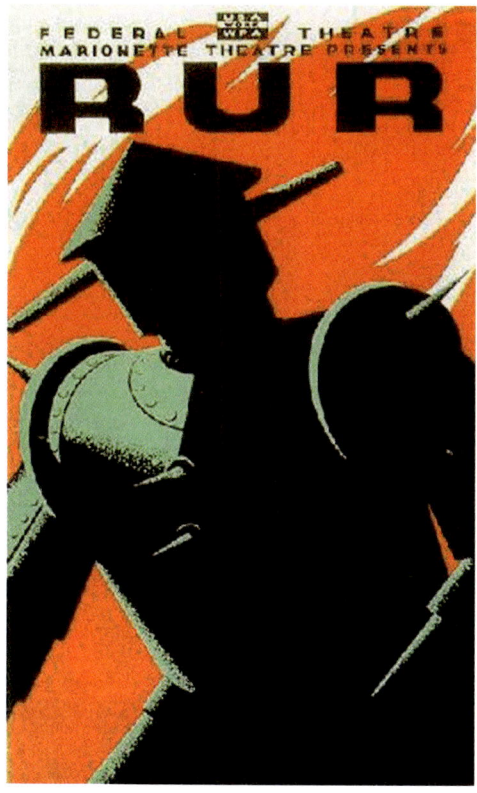

Fig. 14. Cover of R.U.R. by Karel Capek (from http://www.stetson.edu/departments/csata/art).

Robotics also became an integral part of space adventure. Canadarm, a robotic construction unit, became one of the NASA's essential construction tools in outer space (Fig. 16). It has been deployed to repair numerous satellites, telescopes, and shuttles. By the 1990s, NASA started working on their robotic versions of space exploration: rovers, the semiautonomous robotic platforms. The first rover, Sojourner, was launched to Mars in 1996, but it was limited by a short range of movement. By 2004, twin robot rovers were sent to Mars and captured the public's imagination, sending back amazing images of the kilometers of their Mars journey (Fig. 17).

Development of medical science in the late 20th century is marked by a wide incorporation of major technological advancement. It hardly comes as a surprise that robotics made its way into medicine. The inability of the majority of human organs to regenerate has plagued medicine from its

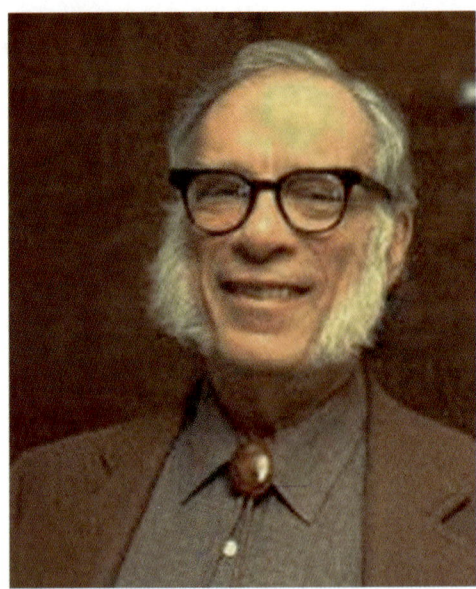

Fig. 15. Portrait of Isaac Asimov (from www.publ.lib.ru).

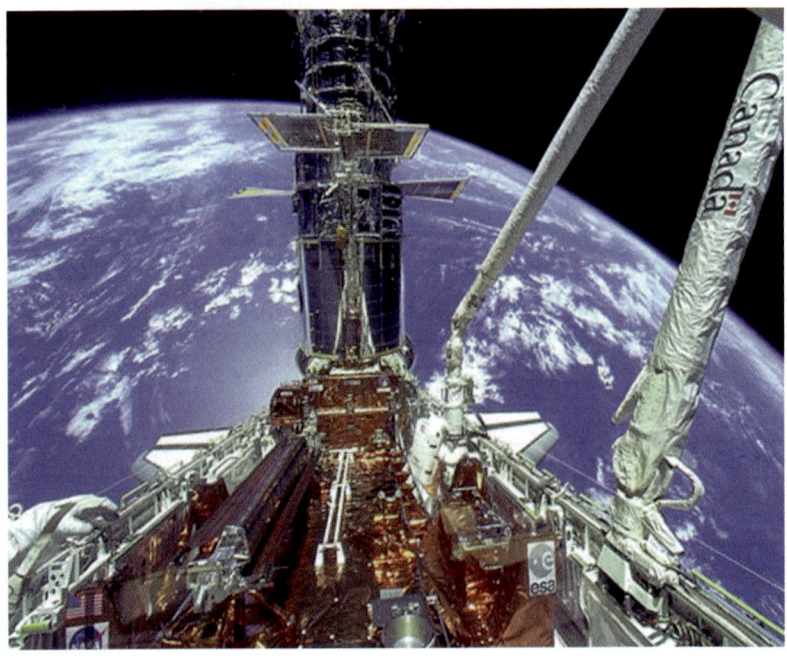

Fig. 16. The Canadarm (from www.nasa.gov).

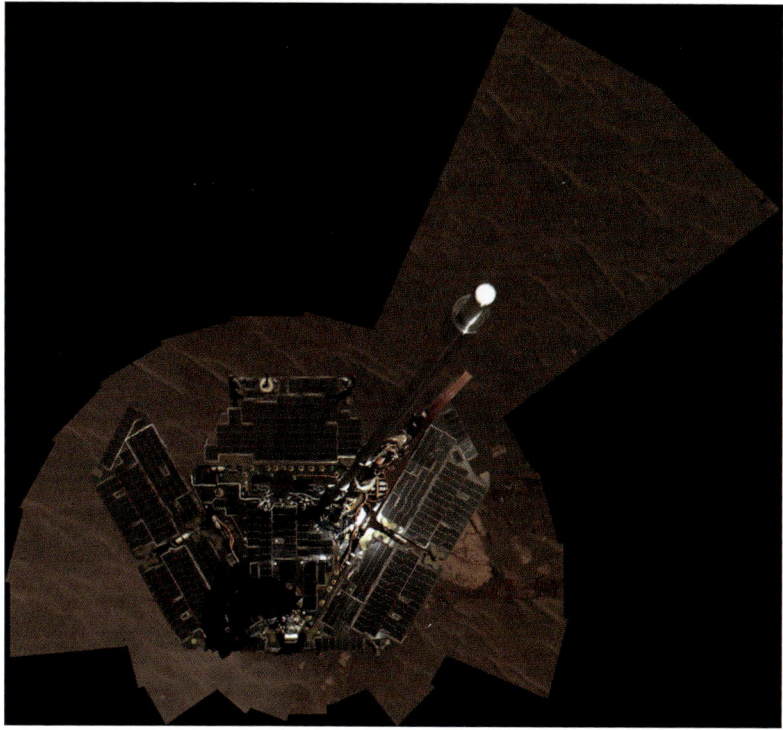

Fig. 17. Mars Rover Opportunity–self portrait (from www.nasa.gov).

beginning. Various primitive limb prosthetics have existed for centuries; however, they were only capable of providing the master with the most basic functions of the lost limb. With rapid advancements in robotics and bioengineering, bionics replacement of human organ became a reality. The first bionic limb was used by Dr. David Gow of the Prosthetic Research and Development Team at Princess Margaret Rose Orthopaedic Hospital of Scotland, UK, in 1998 (Figs. 18–20).

The surgical field traditionally is well attuned with technological developments; therefore, it came as no surprise that robotics made its eventual debut in surgery. The history of surgical robotics begins with Dr. Y. S. Kwoh who first used a robotic system, PUMA 560, to perform neurosurgical biopsies in 1985 (Fig. 21). In 1988, Dr. Davies used the same robotic system for his transurethral resection of prostate. This system eventually led to the development of PROBOT, specifically designed for endoscopic prostate resection (Fig. 22).

Around the same time, another robotic surgical system, ROBODOC, was being developed for application in hip replacement surgery. This

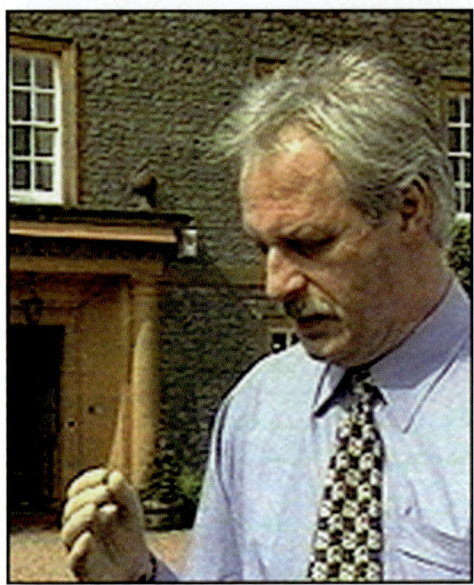

Fig. 18. First bionic arm (from BBC news; news.bbc.co.uk).

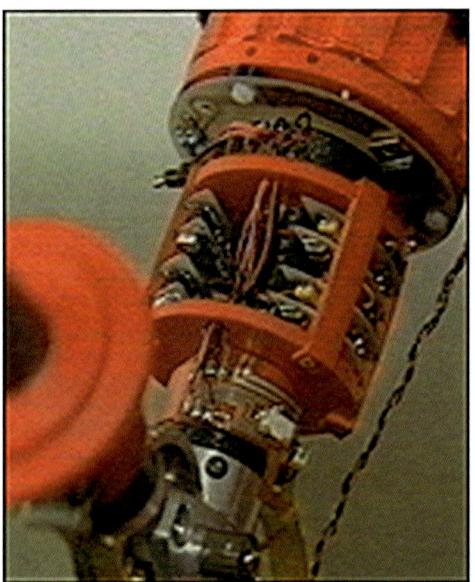

Fig. 19. First bionic arm (from BBC news; news.bbc.co.uk).

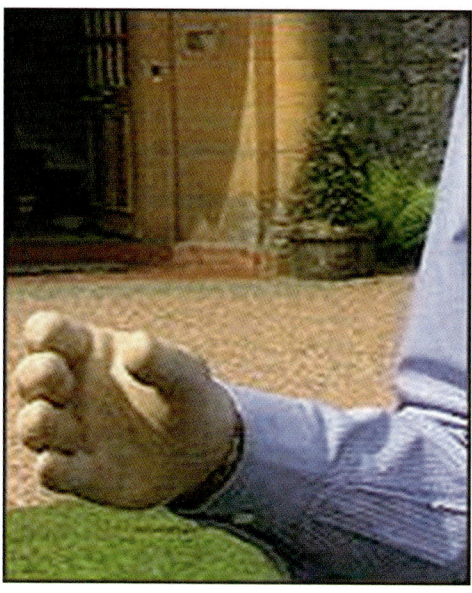

Fig. 20. First bionic arm (from BBC news; news.bbc.co.uk).

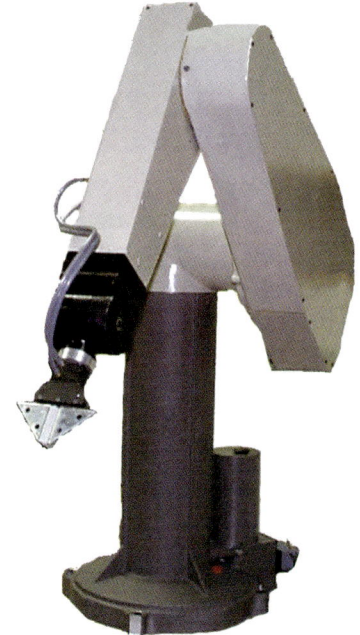

Fig. 21. PUMA 560 robotic system (from http://dma.ing.uniroma1.it/users/delvesco/Web/argo.html)..

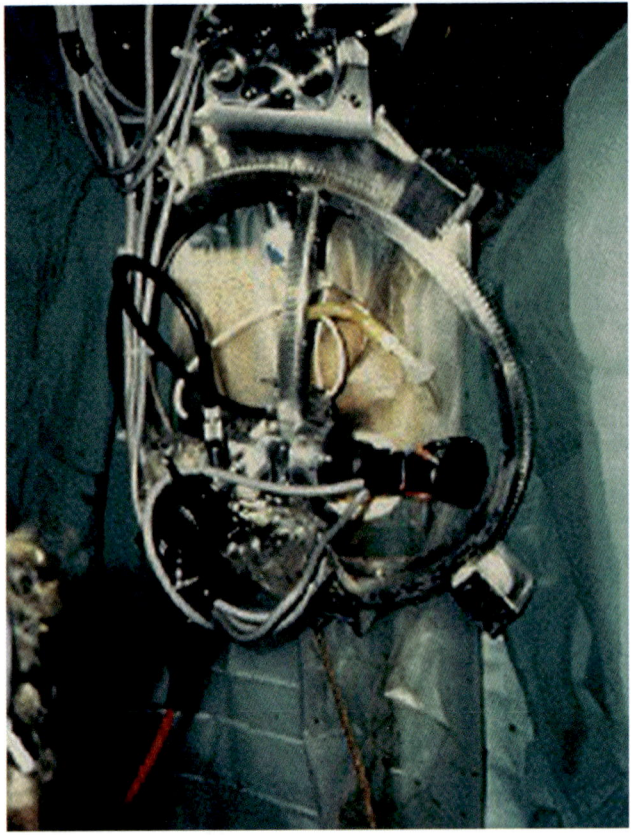

Fig. 22. PROBOT surgical robotic system (from http://www.imperial.ac.uk/ mechatronicsinmedicine/projects/probot/index.html).

system made history in 1992 and became the first surgical robotic system approved by the Food and Drub Administration (FDA).

By the mid-1980s, NASA started to invest into the research of a three-dimensional graphic and audio experience, which later became the basis for the development of virtual reality. The agency was hoping to implement the knowledge it obtained in developing the field of telepresence surgery. Around the same time, Dr. Joseph Rosen, a plastic surgeon from Stanford, together with Dr. Philip Green, started their work on the robotic manipulation system for hand surgery. Later, Dr. Rosen joined the NASA team in exploring the virtual environment and its application to surgery. The original idea was to combine the Stanford experience with robotics and NASA's research with virtual reality. The data glove was developed, which was supposed to track the hand motion of the surgeon at the console and make the robot reproduce the surgeon's movements at the surgical field. Later, the glove was substituted by the handles that are still used for the da Vinci robotic system. The combined work gave birth to the field of telesurgery and became the driving force behind the creation of the surgical robots.

Telesurgery owes its current popularity to several economic and social factors. On the one hand, the U.S. military had a vested interest in the development of a mobile surgical trauma complex for the front line and invested heavily in research and development of telesurgical units. The reasoning behind the investment was obvious. It has been estimated that 90% of combat casualties occur at the battlefield, before the soldier's arrival to the hospital. On the other hand, once wounded soldiers are successfully transported to the Mobile Advance Surgical Hospital (MASH), very few lives are lost thereafter. Therefore, the Pentagon became interested in a surgical system that would provide remote surgical capabilities at the battlefield. The first military prototype was developed by 1994. The robotic arm was mounted in an armored vehicle, Medical Forward Area Surgical Team (MEDFAST). The surgical console was to be installed at the MASH, with surgeon being able to control the robotic arm 10 to 35 km behind the front line. The first remote surgical procedure using MEDFAST was performed by Dr. Jon Bowersox of Stanford, who performed intestinal anastomosis on ex vivo porcine intestine.

Another factor that played a crucial role in acceptance and advancement of telesurgery was more of a societal nature. Obviously, a civilian sector is less in need of a remote surgical system. Furthermore, currently such a system would be in violation of the FDA guidelines, which demand the surgical console and the patient to be in the same operating room during the operative procedure. However, laparoscopic breakthroughs in general surgery, in particular the first laparoscopic cholecystectomy presented in Atlanta, GA, in 1989, fueled the general public's interest of minimally invasive techniques. As laparoscopy matured, its limitations of implementation for challenging surgical techniques became widely recognized. Some of the more prominent limitations included lack of haptic feedback (both force and tactile); two-dimensional video monitoring that complicated visual control; and the need to move the instrument in the opposite direction from the point of interest (so called fulcrum effect), which impeded hand–eye coordination. All of the above-mentioned limitations made challenging surgical procedures, particularly complex anastomotic and microsurgical techniques, unfeasible for laparoscopy. In addition, robotic systems are capable of canceling a physiological tremor of the surgeon via different hardware and software filters, allowing for a precise microsurgical instrumentation.

Also, the amplitude of motion of the surgeon's hands at the controls can be scaled down by the robot, creating the micromotions inside the patient. Enhancement of the laparoscopic capabilities of modern surgical specialties fueled a rapid development of robotic surgical systems.

This book focuses on the implementation of the da Vinci surgical system in urologic practice; therefore, it would only be fair to make a brief overview of its history. The da Vinci Surgical System was designed and produced by the Intuitive Surgical (Figs. 23 and 24). The company was established by Dr. Frederic Moll, and after acquiring the license to the telepresence surgical system, began working on a clinical robotic system. The first prototype was tested in humans in 1997, with the first robotic cholecystectomy performed by Dr. Jacques Himpens of Brussels, Belgium. By then, the system already consisted of the console where

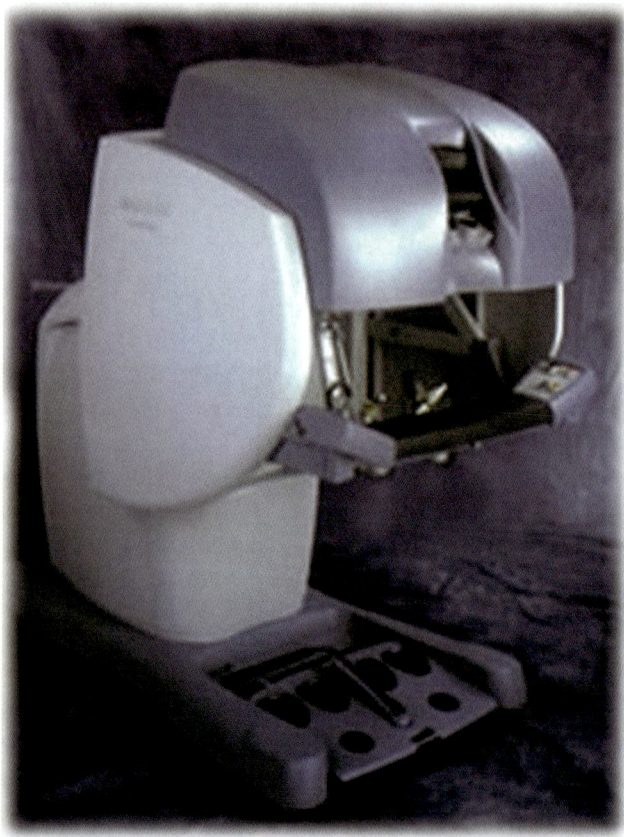

Fig. 23. da Vinci Surgical System console (from http://www.intuitivesurgical. com/).

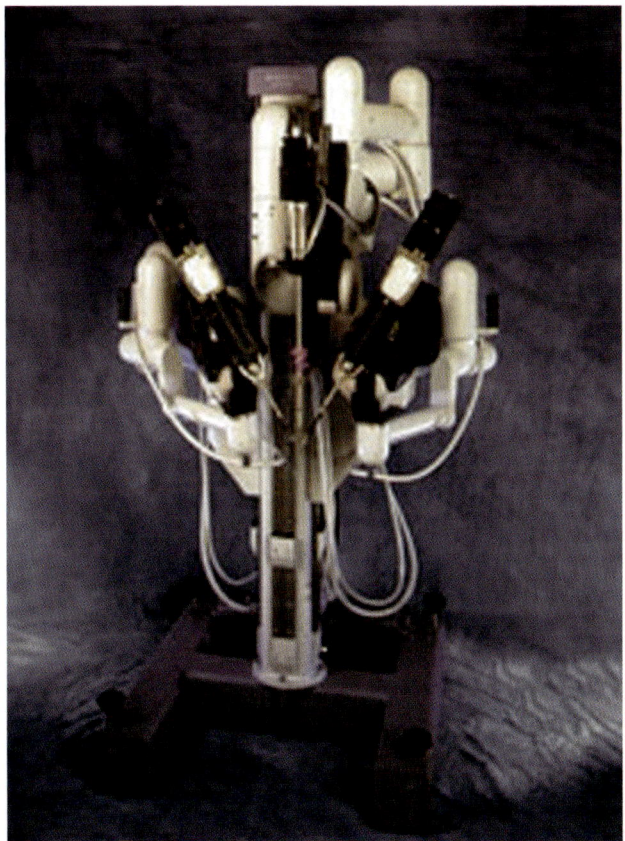

Fig. 24. da Vinci Surgical System patient site cart (from http://www.intuitivesurgical. com/).

the surgeon was performing the operation, and a three-armed telerobot that received the signals from the console and executed surgical manipulations inside the patient's body. The system showed promise, and it had an advantage over the traditional laparoscopic equipment. Unlike laparoscopy, the system had no fulcrum effect created by the body wall and lack of articulation of the instrument. It also had an advantage over laparoscopy in the degrees of freedom (DOF) that it used. DOF is the number of axes of movement of the object. It has been established that to have a full knowledge of the object's movement in three-dimensional (3-D) space, six DOF are required. The six DOF are the sum of the three spatial positions (x, y, and z) and three angles of rotation around the axes (pitch, roll, and yawl). Laparoscopy allows for only four DOF; therefore, it is limited in fine surgical applications. The da Vinci System allows for seven DOF; therefore, it is more suitable for the areas where fine manipulations are required. One of the challenges in the creation of the surgical system was a creation of interface between the wrist of the surgeon and the controls of the machine. After prolonged experimentation, it was determined that the most optimal interaction would be via a tip-to-tip control, where the surgeon's fingers are connected in a virtual manner to the tips of the instruments. The invention enabled the surgeon to implement the familiar hand motions of the open procedures in the robotic cases, unlike pure laparoscopy, where many moves needed to be learned over again, thereby shortening the learning curve of the surgeon. Upon conclusion of a 200-patient trial, the da Vinci Surgical System received FDA approval in July 2000. In December 2002, the FDA approved a new generation of da Vinci telerobots for clinical use in the United States. The next generation system consisted of the four-arm robot, where the fourth arm is identical to the two original instrument arms, and facilitates in retraction. The telescope developed for the da Vinci System is 12 mm in diameter and contains two separate 5-mm telescopes, enabling two separate video signals and providing the surgeon with a 3-D view (Figs. 25 and 26). In the future, Intuitive Surgical is anticipating an addition of a third telescope for a 2-D panoramic perspective. The robotic arm can bend at the elbow, during the motion of the surgical instruments. In addition, most of the instruments articulate at the wrist. The combination of two robotic joints provides the surgeon with seven

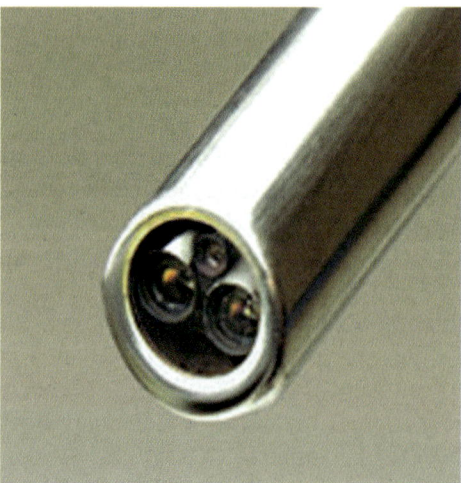

Fig. 25. Endoscope of da Vinci Surgical System (from http://www.intuitivesurgical. com/).

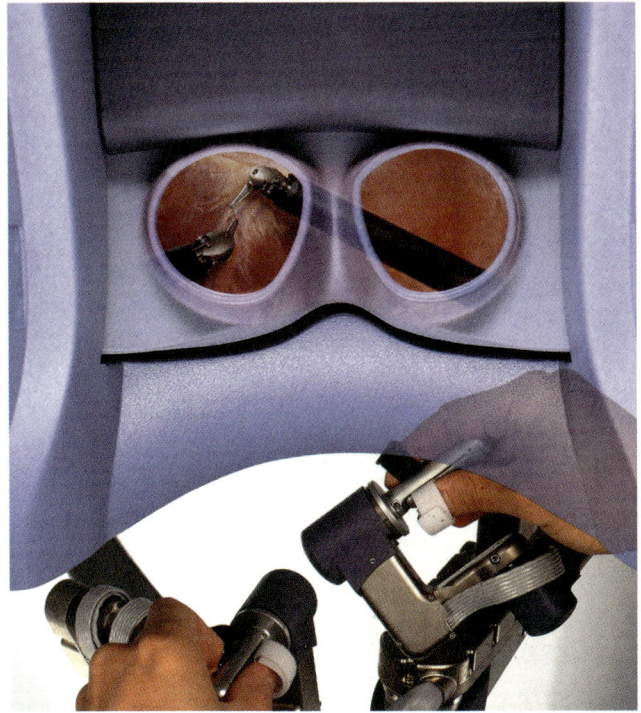

Fig. 26. 3-D visualization of da Vinci Surgical System (from http://www.
intuitivesurgical.com/).

DOF (in and out; elbow up and down; elbow left and right; wrist up
and down; wrist left and right; open and shut; and axial rotation), which
is more than enough to precisely track an object in a 3-D environment
(Fig. 27).

The da Vinci Surgical System also was engineered to provide the
surgeon with a true telepresence experience. As the surgeon looks through
the console, he or she gets instantaneously immersed in a virtual 3-D
operative field, in an essence placing himself or herself inside the patient.
The hood of the console purposefully obscures the peripheral vision,
which is thought to be psychologically advantages, particularly when the
operation is performed remotely.

As Intuitive Surgical was establishing itself in the beginning of 1990s,
another company was emerging into the market. In 1993, a graduate
student at the University of California, Santa Barbara, Yulun Wang,
began developing a new robotic system. He was successful in creation of
the laparoscopic camera holder robot, an Automated Endoscopic System
for Optimal Positioning (AESOP) widely used in laparoscopic surgery

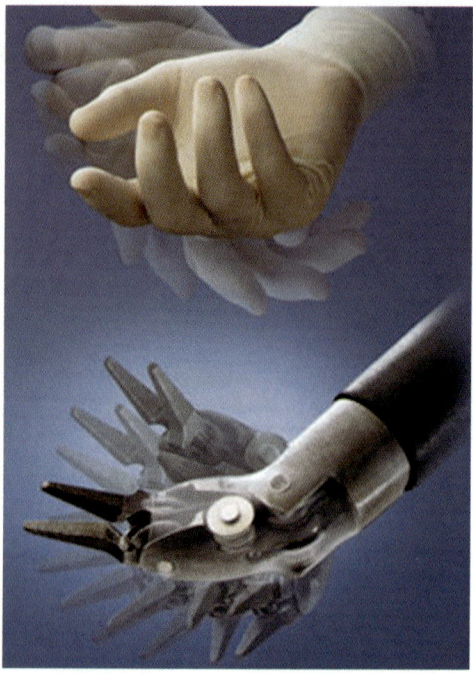

Fig. 27. EndoWrist of da Vinci Surgical System (from http://www.intuitivesurgical. com/).

through the 1990s. AESOP enabled the laparoscopist to perform compli- cated procedures with no help from a specially trained assistant (the camera driver). By 1994, a new company, Computer Motion, Inc., estab- lished by Dr. Wang, emerged in the field of robotics. The company introduced ZEUS Surgical System, which used the same robotic arm as the AESOP and integrated in itself a remote control system (HERMES), also well known to the earlier laparoscopists. There was no attempt made by the company to create a "full emersion experience," the fulcrum effect of laparoscopic surgery was retained, and the 2-D monitoring system. It is beyond the scope of this chapter to discuss the pros and cons of each system in details. It would suffice to mention that the two companies merged in 2003.

The future of robotic surgery is tightly intertwined with the future of healthcare. There are several avenues of progress that have been speculated upon in the literature. Despite the fact that the current FDA requirement is for the surgeon and the patient to be located within the same operating room, if and when this requirement is changed, the robotic system can provide the opportunity for an advanced surgical care at the remote and underserved areas, the same areas that traditionally experience difficulties recruiting qualified medical specialists. The application of telesurgery also widens the teaching capabilities of the robotic surgery by enabling long-distance intraoperative consultations and proctoring.

Another proposed benefit of robotic surgery lies in its potential for a "flawless procedure." As our scanning techniques progress, eventually it will be feasible to reconstruct a 3-D image of the patient's body with a high degree of resolution and detail. Then, a computer interface will be created that will connect the virtual patient with the robotic surgical system and allow the physician to perform "warm-ups" and "practice run" surgeries. The surgeon will be able to rewind and rerun all the steps of the operation until perfection is achieved. Then, the perfected procedure would be recorded and executed in vivo.

Robotic surgery, although still in its infancy, is taking the surgical field by storm. It is still hard to predict whether the current concept of master-slave systems and telerobotics will prevail, or will just serve its purpose as a catalyst for future technological developments. One thing is already obvious, robotics has expanded the horizons of minimally invasive surgery, thrusting the field beyond the limits of human physical abilities. How far it progresses, and whether it reaches beyond human intellectual capabilities, is still the question to be answered.

RESOURCES

1. Hemal AK, Menon M (2004) Robotics in urology. Curr Opin Urol 14:89–93.
2. Lafranco AR et al (2004) Robotic surgery a current perspective. *Ann Surg* 239: 14–21.
3. Ballantyne GH, Moll F (2003) The da Vinci telerobotic surgical system: the virtual operative field and telepresence surgery. Surg Clin North Am 83:1293–1304.
4. Stylopoulos N, Rattner D (2003) Robotics and ergonomics. Surg Clin North Am 83:1321–1337.
5. Stava RM (2003) Robotic surgery: from past to future—a personal journey. Surg Clin North Am 83:1491–1500.
6. History of robotics. www.robotics.megagian.com.
7. The history of robotics by Adam Currie. www.cache.ucr.edu.

II SETUP AND ACCESS

2   Operating Room Setup, Patient and Instrument Preparation

Laura Wisse

1. INTRODUCTION

Urologic procedures in the past decade have taken great strides into advanced laparoscopic procedures. With these advances come planning and implementation of new setups, instruments, and positioning to orchestrate these procedures. Proper planning is essential for efficiency in the operating room. Patient positioning and operating room setup should remain consistent and reproducible according to the specific operation. It is imperative that not only the surgeons are proficient in these areas but also that all the staff members (anesthesiologists, nurses, surgical technicians, equipment technicians, and instrument room technicians) are equally knowledgeable of their specific role in the operation. A collaborative effort makes telerobotic surgery a success.

2. CREATING LAPAROSCOPIC BASKETS

The first question is where to begin. Your institution has just purchased a robotic system, and your surgeons and staff are preparing for training. How do you organize this new acquisition? You may already be doing urologic laparoscopic procedures, so you may have established laparoscopic baskets for specific procedures. If not, creating baskets of laparoscopic instrumentation for basic procedures is a good place to start. When our institution first started out, we created a laparoscopic radical nephrectomy basket and a laparoscopic radical prostate basket. These two baskets are the basis of all urologic telerobotic cases. Your surgeons will need to give input on what instruments they would use for each case and

From: *Current Clinical Urology: Urologic Robotic Surgery*
Edited by: J. A. Stock, M. P. Esposito, and V. J. Lanteri © Humana Press, Totowa, NJ

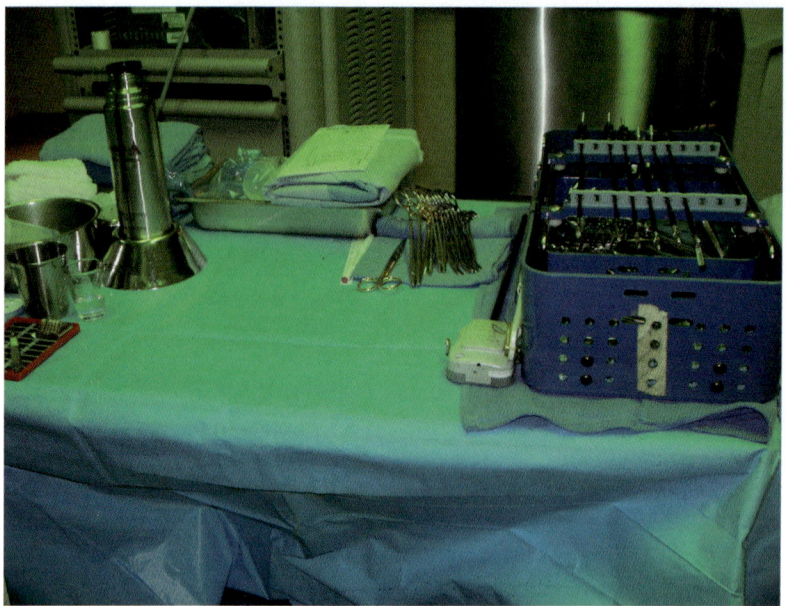

Fig. 1. Back table set up and laparoscopic instrument basket.

confer with everyone and incorporate their needs into one basket. This approach will save time, because you will not be searching for instruments during the case. It will take time to refine your baskets. Instruments that are included in both baskets include laparoscopic ratcheted graspers; laparoscopic rotating graspers; laparoscopic right angles, both 5 and 10 mm; laparoscopic nondisposable clip appliers; laparoscopic scissors; laparoscopic suction cannula; retractors; clamps; forceps; suture scissors; and other instruments to aid in port placement and closure. Create a count sheet for these baskets to ensure that instruments are not missing (Fig. 1).

3. ORGANIZING, CREATING, AND HANDLING ROBOTIC EQUIPMENT

The next step is creating baskets and a system for handling robotic equipment. Creating a robotic accessory basket is a necessity. This basket incorporates all the equipment needed to set up the robot, and it is basic and consistent no matter what robotic case is being done (Fig. 2). Standardizing this basket is also important if your robot is used across different services. In our institution, urology, general, cardiac, gynecology, and thoracic surgery all use the same robotic accessory basket. Robotic instrument arms have been set up in two ways. In our

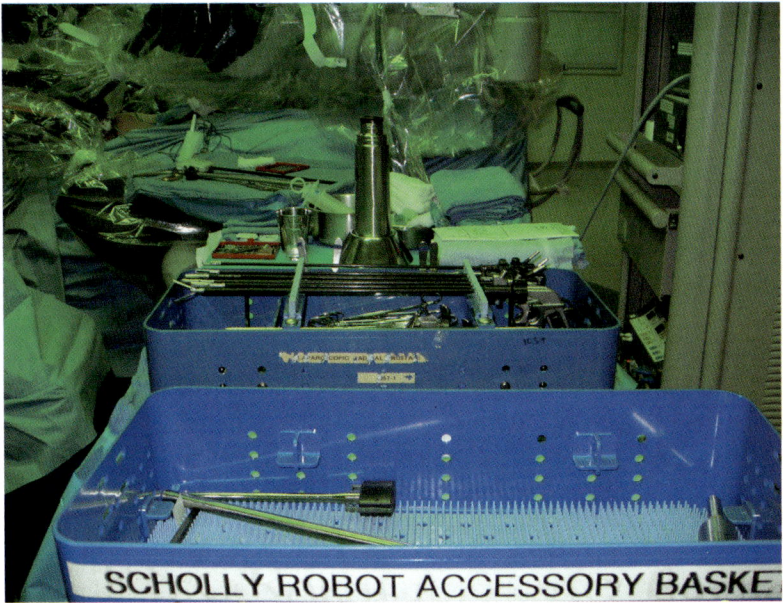

Fig. 2. Back table set up and robot accessory basket.

institution it has been decided to create baskets specific to procedures that include all instrument arms needed for a specific procedure where surgeons are all consistent with the types of instruments they use. Our institution has also chosen to wrap and sterilize each instrument arm individually. The reason behind this decision has to do with each of our surgeons using different instruments to handle the same case. This setup prevents instruments that are not used from getting sterilized unnecessarily. Once you have established the protocol, you need a specific area where all of your robotic baskets and instruments can be organized and stored. A designated area makes it easier to pick for a case, keep inventory on instruments, and prevent loss and breakage of instruments.

At this point, incorporating instrument room techs in the development and upkeep of robotic instruments is essential. They will ultimately be responsible for cleaning and reassembling the baskets and instruments. Robotic instruments require extra time for cleaning. They need to be irrigated through manufacturer's ports, and a thorough cleaning on the outside is necessary to remove gross debris. Ultrasonic cleaning, which uses suction to pull cleaning solution through ports, helps clean out tissue or bodily fluids that have built up. Count sheets for the baskets are key for getting a complete basket returned. Another way to assist the instrument room techs is to provide them with a picture of what is contained in the baskets, as a visual backup to the written count sheet. This approach has helped our institution greatly.

4. CREATING A SURGEON PREFERENCE CARD

Once you have accomplished the task of setting up baskets and instrumentation, the next step is creating a surgeon preference card. You should make the preference card in list form to enable easy reading and picking. Then, determine what supplies would be needed for the cases. There are standardized items that would be common for any procedure whether it is urologic, general, cardiac, or thoracic. These items would include robotic draping, such as instrument arm drapes (two to three depending on how many arms you have or will be using), a camera arm drape, and camera drape. You also need cannula seals for the robotic cannulas (two to three depending on how many arms you have or will be using). A 12-mm disposable trocar is needed for the robotic camera; this trocar may be standard or long length depending on a surgeon's preference. Other disposables for cases depend on the case and the surgeon. Basic items needed for cases common to procedures and surgeons are foleys, syringes, needles, medications, sutures, blades, accessory ports, draping, prep sticks, 4×4s, lap pads, towels, basins, marking pens, insufflation tubing, irrigator, irrigation solution, plum away, thermos seal for scope warmer, laparoscopic pouch, sequentials, padding, razor, tape, lubricant, and draping. Other information included on surgeon preference cards should be glove size, specific robotic instrumentation, medication, cautery settings, room set up, patient positioning preferences, and specific sutures. You can include notes specifying surgeon preferences and needs. All of this information is extremely helpful to those who will be in the room and to those who will be learning these cases. The more specific you can put on the preference card, the easier it is to pick and anticipate needs during the case.

5. SETTING UP A CASE

Now comes the time to put all your preliminary work to use. You have to set up a case. You walk into the room; where do you begin? The first thing you should do is get a feel for the layout of the room. You have to determine the best place to position the robot. You need to take into account what case you are doing and where the surgical arms need to be. If you are doing a prostate, the arms come in between the legs. If you are doing a kidney, the arms come in on the operative side. Then, you must work from this point. The surgical console needs to be in proximity to the arms so as not to stretch the cables from the arms and to allow for the surgeon at the console to have a good view of the surgical field. The video cart needs to go where the surgeon at the field can view it without any obstructions. The video cart also connects to the surgical console, and it cannot be that far from it because of the video cables that run from the video cart to the surgical console. All the cables that connect the arms and video cart to the surgical console must not be walked on, rolled over, or crushed in any way so as to avoid problems with the associated part. Depending on your operating room, you may have booms that incorporate other video equipment if your surgeon chooses to use them for making port placement and closure, which eliminates other carts coming into the room. Otherwise, you need to bring in that video equipment or incorporate the equipment on your robotic video cart. Depending on your operating room, video monitors may be mounted on booms or you may need to bring in a secondary video monitor to provide the whole operating room staff with visual access to the procedure. Ultimately, having equipment booms is ideal to eliminate floor clutter, but they are not always an option. A cautery machine needs to be in proximity to the surgical console to connect the monopolar cord to it and run a bipolar foot pedal to the surgeon at the surgical console. It may be advantageous to add it to your robotic video cart, as we have in our institution, to allow proximity to the console and to decrease floor clutter. You need a standard bed, cushioned stirrups, sequential compression boots, and chair of preference for the surgeon sitting at the surgical console. Also needed is one back table for instrumentation and basic setup. A spinal table is used for the setup of the robotic camera and scope. We use two Mayo stands, one stand for the scrub nurse and a second stand for robotic and laparoscopic instruments for the bedside assistant surgeon. This setup prevents the potential hazard for dropping or contaminating instruments when changing out different robotic instrument arms.

6. POSITIONING THE PATIENT

Now, it is time to incorporate the patient into this setup. The procedure to be performed is involved in how we determine proper patient positioning. For example, with positioning for a robotic assist laparoscopic radical prostatectomy, the patient initially is in a low lithotomy (Fig. 3). The bed has a regular sheet on it, on top of which is placed a gel pad that will be beneath the patient's backside from the shoulders down to the buttocks. Both legs are placed in padded stirrups with additional padding to protect the peroneal nerve (Fig. 4). Both arms are tucked.

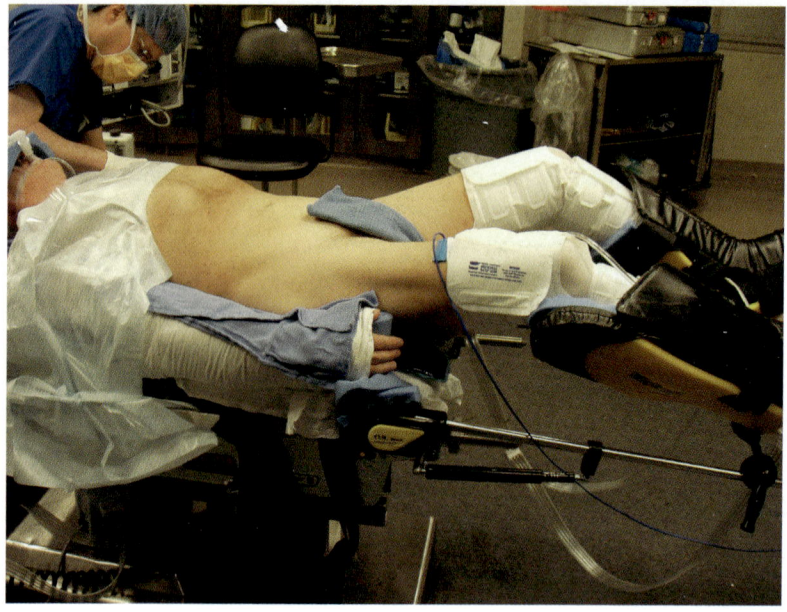

Fig. 3. Patient in Low Lithotomy position showing proper padding of right arm.

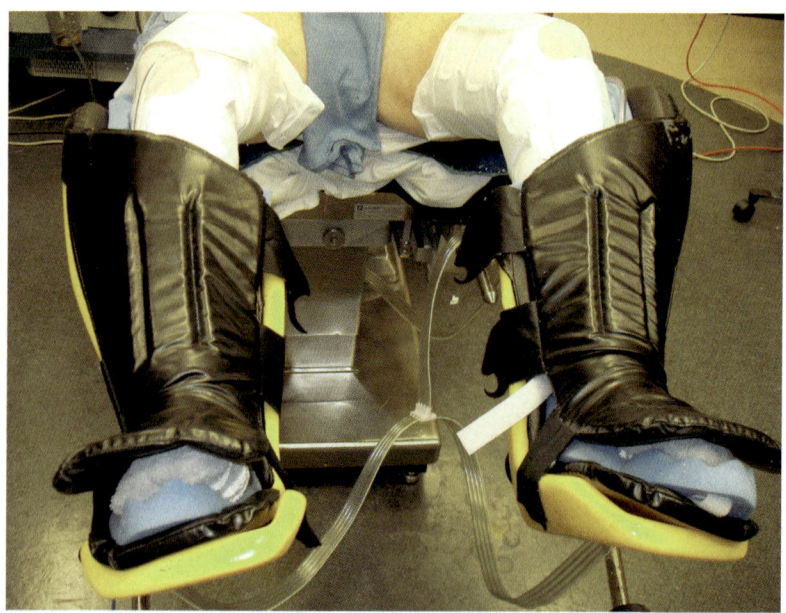

Fig. 4. Patient's arms and legs properly padded.

The right arm gets padding under arm, one folded in hand to promote natural positioning of the fingers, and one pad above the arm, and then the arm is tucked in with draw sheet. The left arm gets one pad under arm and one folded in hand for the same reason we do it for the right arm, and then the arm is tucked in with draw sheet (Fig. 5). The patient then gets put in Trendelenburg position before docking the robot (Fig. 6). Then the robot is brought in and docked on the patient (Fig. 7).

For positioning for robot assist laparoscopic kidney procedures, positioning is different. The patient is in lateral positioning, and depending on your surgeon's preference, positioning devices can vary. Some surgeons prefer using a beanbag, some a gel pad over bean bag, and others just the gel pad. The same goes for the arm; the one arm that is on the patient's down side is on an arm board, and the other arm also can vary with the positioning devices used. Some surgeons like to use a Krause arm support, whereas others use pillows or blankets. Which ever you choose, securing the arm is essential. Leg positioning is standardized; the lower leg is bent, the upper leg is straight, and pillows are placed between the two legs for cushioning. Also, ulnar pads are placed under the foot to cushion it against the table (Fig. 8).

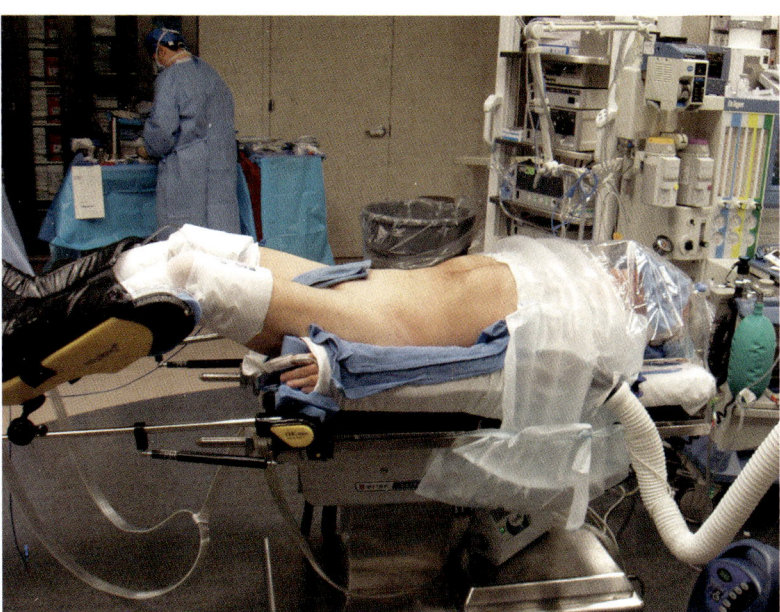

Fig. 5. Patient's arms and legs properly padded.

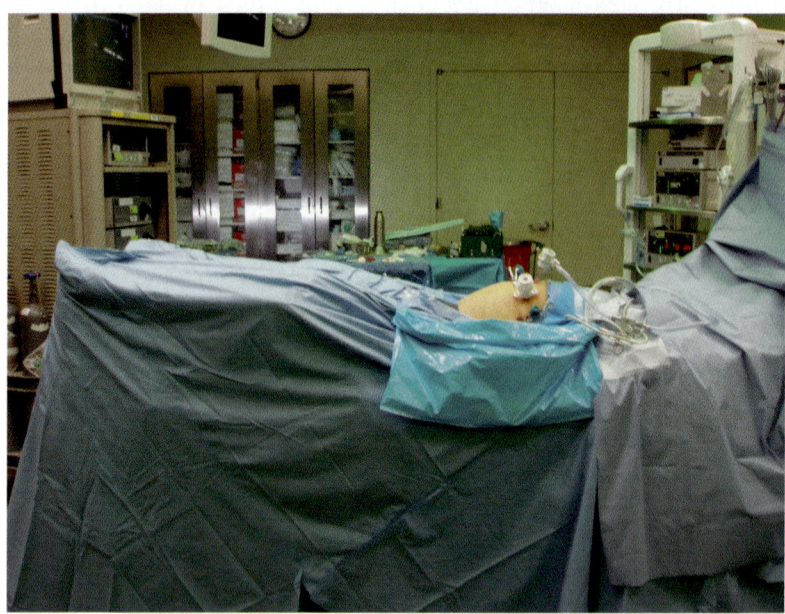

Fig. 6. Patient placed in Low Lithotomy and Trendlenberg position before docking the robot.

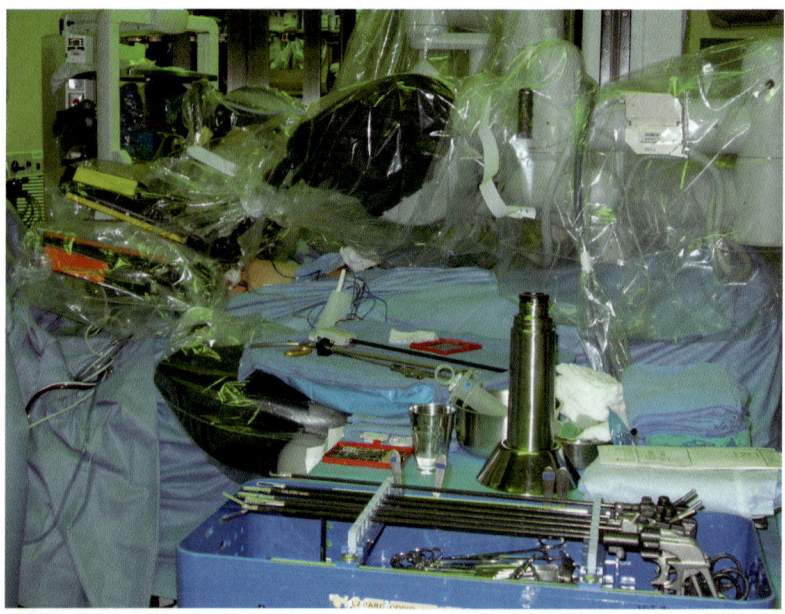

Fig. 7. Robot docked on patient.

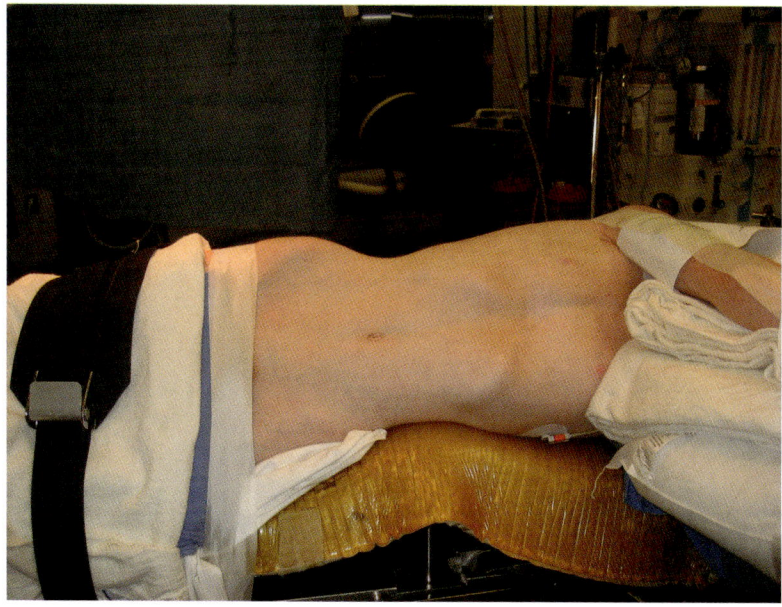

Fig. 8. Positioning of patient for Kidney procedure.

As you do more cases and develop your own preferences, you will see what is needed and what changes could be made to ensure a smooth case for each surgeon. Always adjust your preference cards to reflect any changes to ensure there is no wasting of disposables and time.

3 Port Placement and Exit

Rahuldev S. Bhalla

1. INTRODUCTION

The majority of urologic laparoscopic procedures are performed via the transperitoneal approach. The peritoneal cavity can be reliably entered and distended. It provides a large working space, and in addition, most urologists are comfortable with the anatomy. Patient preparation for our program includes a bowel prep the night before surgery, with one bottle of magnesium citrate and a clear liquid diet. If a radical prostatectomy is to be performed, we also give a Fleets enema the night before surgery.

All patients receive general endotracheal anesthesia an oral gastric tube and a Foley catheter before positioning. Care is taken to pad all pressure points and to secure the patient to the table. Appropriate antibiotics are given perioperatively, and the field is prepped widely in the event an open incision has to be made.

2. VERESS NEEDLE ACCESS (CLOSED TECHNIQUE)

The most commonly used technique is with the Veress needle. The Veress needle is a 14-guage needle with a spring-loaded protective tip that allows for closed insufflation of the abdomen. Disposable and nondisposable metal Veress needles are available commercial in different lengths, i.e., long for obese patients, short for thin or pediatric patients. Before using veress needle, it should always be checked for its patency and spring action. The most commonly used site for the introduction of the Veress needle is the superior or inferior margin of the umbilicus. The reason this site is chosen is because the abdominal wall is two layers thick, with only fascia and peritoneum. Placement of the needle is a blind procedure with the potential for injury to the underlying structures. If the patient has undergone prior surgery, this technique should be avoided.

From: *Current Clinical Urology: Urologic Robotic Surgery*
Edited by: J. A. Stock, M. P. Esposito, and V. J. Lanteri © Humana Press, Totowa, NJ

The patient should be placed into a slight Trendelenburg position to help lift the small intestines out of the pelvis. A small incision is made at the superior or inferior margin of the umbilicus based on patient anatomy and proposed procedure. The anterior abdominal wall can be elevated by grasping the periumbilical area with sharp towel clamps. The Veress needle is held like a dart (Fig. 1). The angle of the needle should be in the direction of the pelvis. When entering the peritoneum, two distinct "pops" should be felt. The first is when the needle transverses the fascia, and the second is when the needle transverses the peritoneum.

Once the needle is in the peritoneum, we perform confirmation tests:

1. Aspiration to check for fluid or sucus.
2. Drop test: Take a syringe with 2 cc of saline and place a drop inside the hub of the needle and lift on the abdominal wall. If the needle is in proper position, the drop will enter the abdomen.
3. Insufflate at low rate and if the pressures remain <8 mmHg, the needle is in the proper position.
4. Lift the anterior abdominal wall and notice a pressure drop.

After ensuring the needle is in the proper position, insufflate the abdomen with CO_2 at low flow (2-3 l/min). The initial pressures should be <8 mmHg. After 1 liter of gas is insufflated the flow is increased to high

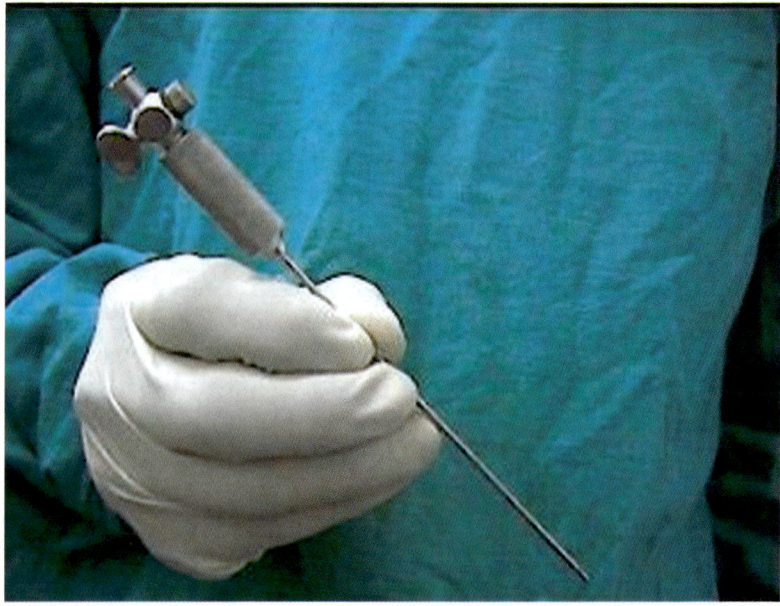

Fig. 1. Veress needle.

flow (>15 l/min). Maximum intra-abdominal pressure is set to 15 mmHg. A high intra-abdominal pressure at low flow suggests that improper needle placement.

After the pneumoperitoneum is established, the Veress needle is removed and the primary trocar is introduced. A 10/12-mm trocar is used in adults to allow passage of the laparoscope. This trocar designation refers to the size of the instruments that can be passed through the sheath, not to the width of the trocar. There are several types of trocars from sharp to blunt tip to optical visualization. There are >20 manufacturers and 100 different brands *(1)*. The incision site for the Veress needle should be enlarged and the subcutaneous tissue spread to the fascia using a hemostat.

The proper technique for inserting a trocar is with a constant steady pressure with a gently twisting motion. The index finger should be held along the shaft to control the trocar movement upon penetration (Fig. 2). The abdominal wall should be lifted and stabilized by towel clamps. The trocar should be directed toward the pelvis. Entry into the peritoneum is indicated with a decrease in resistance. Most disposable sharp trocars have a safety shield that will deploy once resistance has decreased. The sharp obturator is removed, and briefly opening the stopcock will cause a rush of gas, suggesting correct placement.

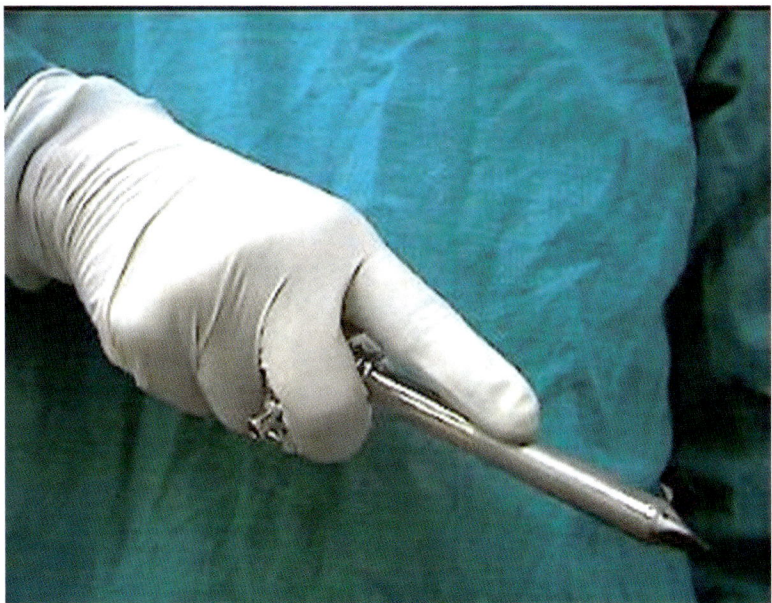

Fig. 2. Correct hand positioning for trocar placement.

The chance of serious injury is greater when inserting the primary trocar compared with a Veress needle secondary to the size of the trocar. The CO_2 insufflator is connected to the stopcock on the trocar. The laparoscope should be warmed and placed through this port. A complete visual inspection of the abdomen is mandatory after placement of the primary trocar regardless of the technique.

3. HASSON TECHNIQUE (OPEN TECHNIQUE)

Hasson technique is our preferred access technique for all patients. This technique allows standardization of all our instruments and trocars, and it eliminates a blind primary trocar placement. The advantage is that of entry into the peritoneal cavity under direct vision, thereby minimizing the risk of injury and extraperitoneal insufflation. We make an initial vertical incision, either supra or infraumbilical based on patient habitus and procedure. This incision is carried down through the subcutaneous tissue with electrocautery. The fascia is identified and cleared off. An incision is made through the fascia with a knife on a long handle. A 0-Vicryl suture is then placed through both edges of the fascia as stay sutures. This procedure serves two purposes. First, it allows us to secure the Hasson trocar to the abdominal wall; and second, it aids in closure. After the stay sutures are placed, the peritoneum is scored with a 15 blade knife, and the peritoneum is entered. The Hasson trocar (Fig. 3) is placed in and secured with the preplaced stay sutures. The sleeve of the trocar

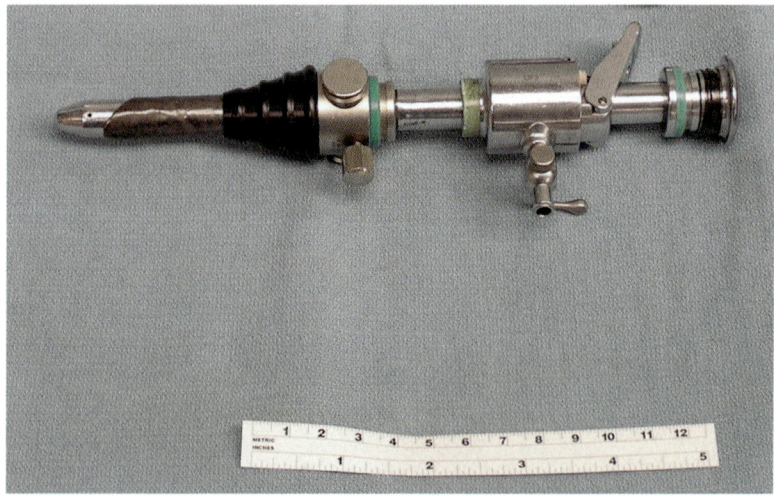

Fig. 3. Hasson trocar.

is wrapped with petroleum jelly gauze to prevent leakage of insufflated gas around the trocar.

The abdomen is then insufflated with CO_2 at low flow (2–3 l/min). Once again, the initial pressures should be <8 mmHg. After 1 to 1.5 liters has been insufflated into the abdomen, the flow should be increased to 15–20 l/min. The maximum intraabdominal pressure should be set to 15 mmHg. Once again, the intraabdominal contents should be visually inspected for any injury.

4. SECONDARY PORT PLACEMENT

Trocar sites and sizes are selected based on the procedure to be performed, patient anatomy, and surgeon preference. At least one 10-mm trocar is placed to allow for the passage of larger instruments. Trocar placement for specific procedures is discussed in the appropriate chapters.

The placement of the working ports can be monitored both internally and externally. The safety of placing these ports is increased because of direct visualization. After the appropriate site is located externally, we confirm this internally by palpation with an index finger. The site is evaluated to confirm that there are no underlying vessels or bowel. Next, a 25 gauge "finder" needle is used to confirm the intraabdominal placement of the port. After this is completed, a skin incision is made parallel to Langer's lines. The skin incision should be large enough to accommodate the trocar and remove the skin as a point of resistance during trocar insertion but not large enough to allow gas leakage. Spread the subcutaneous tissue with a hemostat or tonsil clamp to the level of the fascia. The trocar should be introduced with the same technique as described for the primary trocar except that the intraabdominal progress can be monitored via the laparoscope. In general, the secondary trocars should be placed in the midline or lateral to the rectus muscle to avoid bleeding from the muscle or injury to the epigastric vessels.

5. EXTRAPERITONEAL/RETROPERITONEAL LAPAROSCOPY

The extraperitoneal approach has been used in patients to reduce the risk of visceral and vascular injury. Prolonged ileus may be less common, and fluid may be more easily contained. Herniation through trocar sits, postoperative ileus, and adhesions may be less than that of the transperitoneal approach. The extraperitoneal approach may be limited by prior surgical procedures or inflammatory processes that may obliterate the potential space. The limited retroperitoneal working space may make placement of the trocars more difficult as well as limiting the removal of large masses. There also may be more CO_2 absorption in the extraperitoneal space *(2)*.

Simple extraperitoneal insufflation causes the gas to track along fascial planes and not to develop the space. Balloon dissection of the extraperitoneal space is key to performing any extraperitoneal procedure. Gaur was the first to describe balloon distention of the extraperitoneal space by using a simple device consisting of a sterile glove finger mounted on a red rubber catheter *(3)*. Currently, there are several trocar-mounted balloons available.

Initially, a 2-cm incision is made at the tip of the 12th rib. This incision is carried down to the retroperitoneal space. The index finger should be used to develop the space initially and sweep the peritoneum anteriorly. The balloon is lubricated and placed toward the lower pole of the kidney. The balloon is kept inflated for 5 min to facilitate hemostasis. After balloon removal, a Hasson blunt-tipped trocar is inserted and secured by the trocar's retention mechanism. Visualization of the psoas confirms proper balloon dilation. The secondary ports are placed at the posterior and anterior axillary lines at the discretion of the surgeon.

6. TROCAR REMOVAL AND PORT CLOSURE

At the end of the procedure, the pressure should be lowered to 5 mmHg or less to observe for any bleeding that may be tamponaded by the pneumoperitoneum. Trocar sites should be examined for bleeding, and

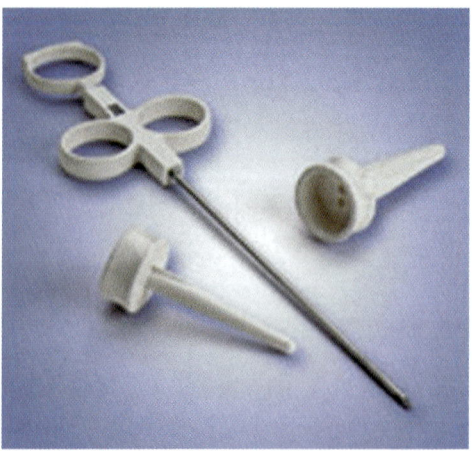

Fig. 4. Carter-Thomason device.

they should be removed under direct visualization. During removal, bowel can be entrapped. Ports that are 10 mm or larger require fascial suturing using a Norwalk, CT, or the Carter-Thomason closure (Fig. 4) device (Inlet Medical, Eden Prairie, MN). A free 0-Vicryl is passes percutaneously and grasped with either device and withdrawn.

7. COMPLICATIONS

Between 1997 and mid-2002, the Food and Drug Administration received >1,300 laparoscopic trocar-associated injury reports, including reports of approximately 30 deaths (1). Most injuries were associated with primary trocar placement. There is an increase in morbidity and mortality when the injury is not initially recognized and treated.

The incidence of major vascular injury is around 0.02 to 0.24% (4). Most of these injuries, if not all, occurred using the closed technique in an elective setting. These injuries generally involve the aorta or the iliac vessels, but they can involve any other major blood vessel. Diagnosis and immediate repair are the mainstays of treatment. Generally, most of these injuries are converted to an open laparotomy.

Bowel injury occurs in 0.03 to 0.15% irrespective of the technique used to access the peritoneum. Most of these injuries can be repaired laparoscopically. If initially missed, persistent tachycardia may be the earliest sign in the immediate postoperative period of enteral perforation. Tachycardia will be followed by low-grade temperature and persistent leukocytosis and continued postoperative pain beyond what should be normally expected (5).

Trocar injury is a recognized complication of laparoscopic and robotic surgery. There is no foolproof method of creating pneumoperitoneum, and constant vigilance is always required to promptly recognize and address these injuries.

REFERENCES

1. Fuller J, Scott W, Ashar B, Corrado J (2003) Laparoscopic trocar injuries: a report from the Food and Drug Administration (FDA) Center for Devices and Radiologic Health (CDRH) Systematic Technology Assessment of Medical Products (STAMP) committee. Food and Drug Administration, Rockville, Maryland.
2. Mullet CE, Viale JP, Sagnard PE et al (1993) Pulmonary CO_2 elimination during surgical procedure using intra- or extraperitoneal CO_2 insufflation. Anesth Analg 76:622.
3. Gaur DD (1992) Laparoscopic operative retroperitoneoscopy: use of a new device. J Urol 148:1137.
4. Catarci M, Carlini M, Gentileschi P, Santoro E (2001) Major and minor injuries during the creation of pneumoperitoneum. Surg Endosc 15:566–569.
5. Gaar E (2004) Errors in laparoscopic surgery. J Surg Oncol 88:153–160.

III Robotic Laparoscopic Procedures

4

Robotic Transperitoneal Four Arm Laparoscopic Radical Prostatectomy: Points of Technique

Sagar R. Shah and Vipul R. Patel

1. INTRODUCTION

Prostate cancer accounts for 33% of all newly diagnosed cancers in men. It was estimated that in 2004 in the United States, the incidence of prostate cancer was 230,000 cases with approximately 29,900 deaths from the disease *(1)* Approximately 77,000 radical prostatectomies are performed yearly for the treatment of prostate cancer. Currently, the gold standard for treatment is open radical retropublic prostatectomy (RRP), which has demonstrated a reduction in disease specific mortality for patients with localized prostate cancer *(2)*. However, this treatment option is invasive and can potentially lead to significant morbidity in terms of pain, blood loss, and prolonged recovery. As such, patients and surgeons alike have sought out less invasive surgical options. One such alternative is robotically assisted laparoscopic radical prostatectomy (RALP).

Initial reports of the use of telerobotic surgical systems to facilitate performance of laparoscopic radical prostatectomy (LRP) were presented in 2001 by Abbou *(3)*, Pasticier *(4)*, Binder *(5)*, and Rassweiler *(6)*. Robotic assistance with the da Vinci Surgical System (Intuitive Surgical, Sunnyvale, CA) has been reported to aid in the performance of laparoscopic prostatectomy secondary to the following: (1) restoration of depth perception and improved vision due to 10× magnification along with three-dimensional vision; (2) wristed miniature instrumentation with restoration of 7° of surgical freedom; (3) tremor filtering and scaling of movements, which aids in fine dissection and precise suturing; (4)

From: *Current Clinical Urology: Urologic Robotic Surgery*
Edited by: J. A. Stock, M. P. Esposito, and V. J. Lanteri © Humana Press, Totowa, NJ

intuitive finger-controlled movement; and (5) improved ergonomics and relaxed surgeon working position, providing for reduced surgeon fatigue *(3–13)*. It has been reported that due to these advantages over conventional laparoscopy, robotic assistance has accelerated learning in the laparoscopically naïve surgeon and has reduced the learning curve to achieve 4-h proficiency down to 12–18 cases without significant outcome variation *(13–16)*.

2. INDICATIONS AND CONTRAINDICATIONS

The indications for robot-assisted laparoscopic prostatectomy via the transperitoneal approach have been described to be similar to those of open and laparoscopic prostatectomy. Patients should have localized prostate cancer, biologically significant disease, and life expectancy >10 years *(7,17)*. It is often easier to perform RALP compared with conventional RRP in patients that have undergone prior laparoscopic inguinal herniorrhaphy *(17)*. Also, it is thought that robotic prostatectomies allow patients with increased comorbidities to undergo surgery whereas otherwise they would have been considered poor candidates for the open surgical approach. Relative contraindication to RALP is weight >300 pounds, body mass index >40, previously ruptured viscera, history of peritonitis, and prior pelvic radiation therapy.

3. POINTS OF TECHNIQUE

3.1. Operating Room Setup

It is recommended that before the patient is placed on the operating room table the robot and the operative table should be aligned in a straight line to the foot of the bed. This is to facilitate easy positioning of the robot between the patient's legs. The assistant and surgical technician should be placed on the right s of the patient and the fourth arm positioned to the left side (Fig. 1).

3.2. Patient Positioning

The patient is positioned supine on a padded beanbag in low lithotomy by using Allen stirrups. All pressure points are padded. The legs are spread apart to allow the robot to come in between, and the patient is then strapped into position (Fig. 2).

3.3. Intra-Abdominal Access and Trocar Placement

Access to the pelvic cavity can be preperitoneal or transperitoneal. Our preference has been the transperitoneal approach due to the larger

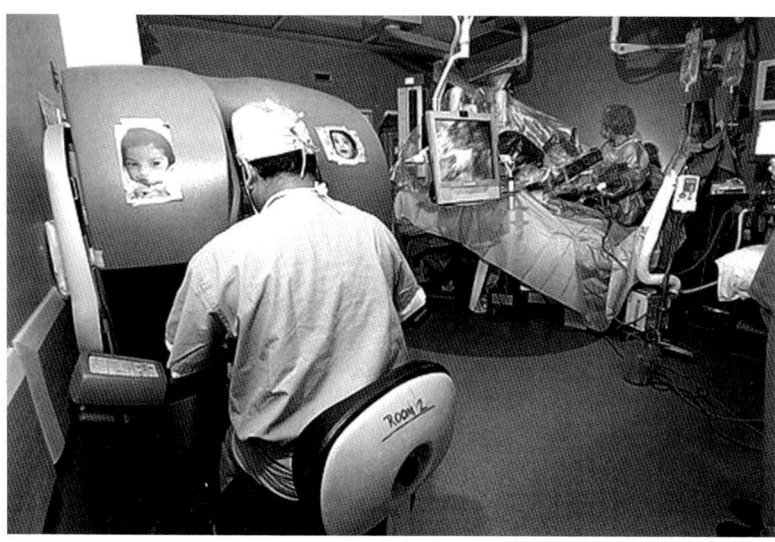

Fig. 1. Operating room setup. Surgeon operates da Vinci Surgical System from console. The surgical assistant and scrub nurse are both positioned to the right of the patient. Patient shown in Trendelenburg position.

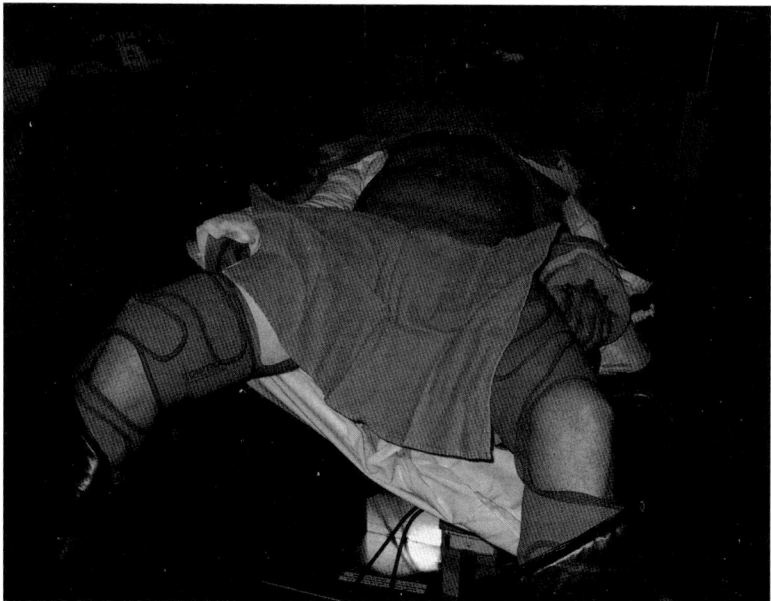

Fig. 2. Patient positioning. Patient is placed in low lithotomy, with legs spread apart to allow docking of robot in between the legs. Patient's arms are carefully padded, tucked and placed to the side.

working space. Some of the potential advantages to the preperitoneal approach are decreased incidence of bowel injury, ileus, or urinoma formation. However, in our transperitoneal series we have not experienced any significant incidence of these complications, and we have opted for the larger working spaces. The intra-abdominal access is obtained by either a Veress needle or a Hasson technique. Once access is obtained, the abdomen is insufflated with CO_2 to 15 mmHg. Under direct vision, the peripheral trocars are placed as shown in Fig. 3. Two 12-mm, three 8-mm da Vinci trocars, and one 5-mm trocar are used. The assistant trocars are placed on the periphery to allow easy access and to avoid the bulky arms of the robot. The patient is then placed in a steep 30° Trendelenburg position, and the robot is docked between the patient's legs.

Trocar Placement

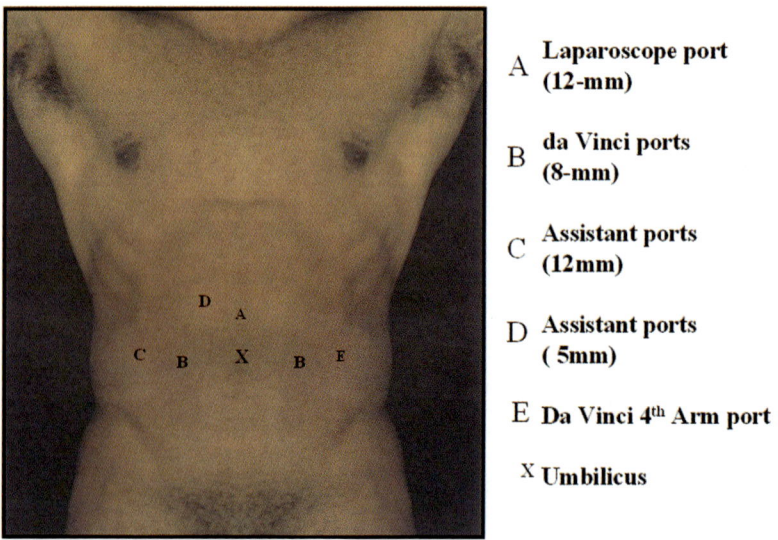

A **Laparoscope port (12-mm)**

B **da Vinci ports (8-mm)**

C **Assistant ports (12mm)**

D **Assistant ports (5mm)**

E **Da Vinci 4th Arm port**

X **Umbilicus**

Fig. 3. Trocar positioning. **A** 12-mm port placed just cephalad to the umbilicus for robotic camera. **B** Two 8-mm da Vinci ports are placed inferior and lateral to umbilicus and approximately 8–9 cm away and inferior to the camera port. **C** 12-mm assistant port is placed laterally between the right ASIS and the right robotic trocar. **D** 5-mm assistant port is placed lateral and cranial to the camera port with adequate spacing to avoid interference from or with camera port. **E** The fourth arm is placed on the left between the ASIS and the left robotic trocar.

3.4. *Transperitoneal Robotic Prostatectomy*

3.4.1. STEP 1: INCISION OF PERITONEUM AND ENTRY INTO RETROPUBIC SPACE (FIG. 4)

The procedure is begun by using a 0° binocular lens, plasma-kinetic (PK) dissector, and monopolar scissors. The peritoneum is incised to enter the retropubic space of Retzius. The boundaries are the pubic bone superiorly, the median umbilical ligaments laterally, and the vas deferens inferolaterally. Maximal exposure is essential to facilitate the procedure.

3.4.2. STEP 2: INCISION OF ENDOPELVIC FASCIA AND LIGATION OF DORSAL VENOUS COMPLEX (FIGS. 5 AND 6)

The endopelvic fascia is then opened immediately lateral to the reflection of the puboprostatic ligaments bilaterally and the levator fibers are pushed off the prostate until the dorsal venous complex is visualized. The dorsal vein is then suture ligated with a 0-Caprosyn on a CT-1 needle by using the robotic needle drivers. A suspension stick is then placed from the public bone to the dorsal venous complex with monocryl 1 on a CT-1 needle to stabilize the periurethral complex.

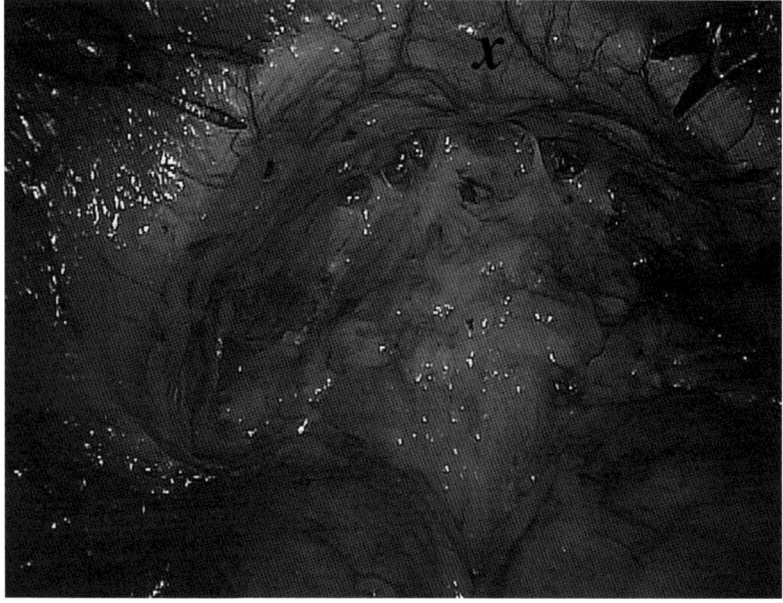

Fig. 4. Retropubic space. The retropubic space is identified. Showing the landmarks of the public bone (*X*), levators, and prostate.

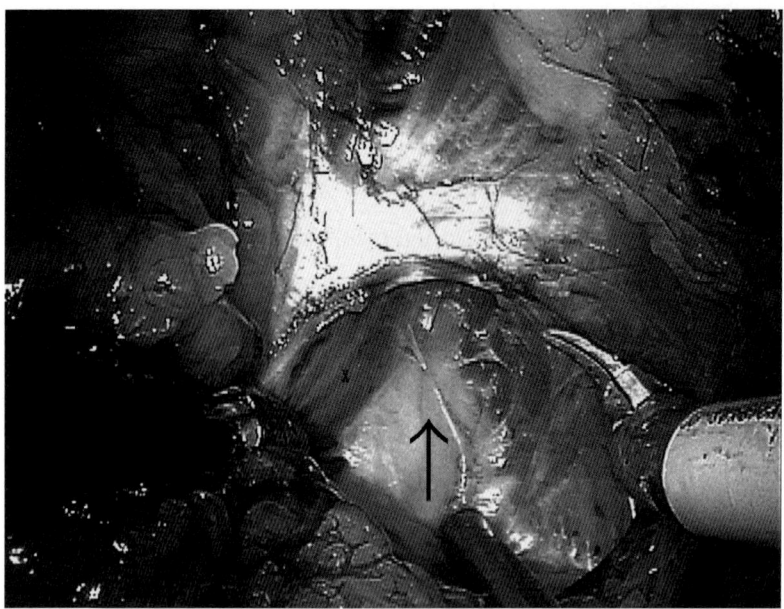

Fig. 5. Incision of endopelvic fascia. The endopelvic fascia is opened with robotic scissors. *X*, prostate. *Arrow*, perirectal fat in plane below opened endopelvic fascia.

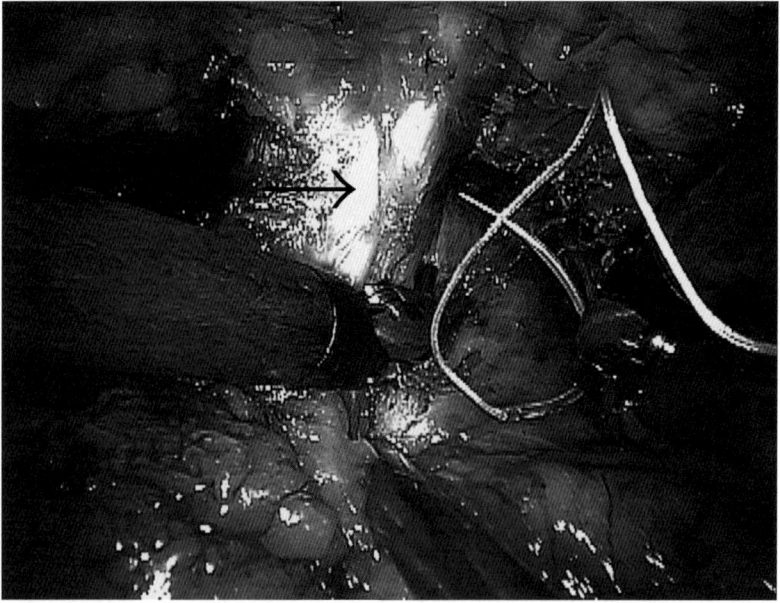

Fig. 6. Suture ligature of dorsal venous (DVC) complex. The DVC (*arrow*) is identified and ligated.

3.4.3. STEP 3: ANTERIOR BLADDER NECK DISSECTION

The laparoscope is then changed to a 30° down lens for the bladder neck dissection. Visual clues are of supreme importance and are used to guide the plane of dissection. The Foley catheter is pulled on to help define the bladder neck. If the Foley deviates laterally, this usually indicates the presence of a median lobe. The bladder neck is further identified by the cessation of fat extending from the bladder. The robotic arms also provide visual and some sensory feedback as the instruments are used to appreciate the consistency of the bladder and prostate (Double pinch maneuver). The bladder is dissected off the prostate in the midline using the sweeping motion of the monopolar scissors. Once the anterior urethra is divided, the Foley catheter is retracted out of the bladder in an upward direction using the fourth arm, exposing the posterior bladder neck.

3.4.4. STEP 4: POSTERIOR BLADDER NECK

The posterior bladder neck dissection is generally considered to be the most challenging aspect of the operation for the novice robotic surgeon. The problem lies in the difficulty appreciating the tissue plane between bladder and prostate posteriorly and the direction and depth of dissection necessary to locate the seminal vesicles.

The recommended approach is as follows: After incision of the anterior bladder neck any remaining peripheral bladder attachments should be divided to flatten out the area of the posterior bladder neck and allow precise visualization and dissection of the posterior plane. The posterior bladder neck should be incised full thickness at the precise junction between the prostate and the bladder. Once this is performed, the lip of posterior bladder neck is grasped with the PK dissector and used for gentle traction to visualize the natural plane between the prostate and bladder inferiorly. The dissection is directed downward and slightly back towards the bladder to visualize the seminal vesicles. It is of importance to avoid dissecting forward toward the prostate, because there is a possibility of getting into prostatic tissue and missing the seminal vesicles completely. An excellent clue as to the correct surgical plane is the presence of a plane of fat between the prostate and bladder. Bladder fibers can also help guide the dissection.

3.4.5. STEP 5: SEMINAL VESICLE DISSECTION

Once the initial portion of the posterior dissection is complete and the bladder has been dissected off, the prostate, the vasa and seminal vesicles can be identified. The thin fascial layer over the seminal vesicles and vasa should be opened to free up the structures for retraction. The fourth arm is used to retract the vasa superiorly. Both vasa are then incised, and the inferior portion of the vas is retracted by the assistant. The vas is then followed posteriorly to expose the tips of the seminal vesicles. Small perforating vessels are clipped and divided. Both seminal vesicles are delivered in a similar manner. It is of supreme importance to dissect the seminal vesicles fully to the base to allow for the appropriate retraction of the prostate and to correctly visualize the plane of dissection between the prostate and the rectum.

3.4.6. STEP 6: DENONVILLIERS' FASCIA AND POSTERIOR DISSECTION

A rectal bougie can be placed to aid in the identification and dissection of this plane. The rectal bougie is manipulated to visualize the arc that represents the correct plane between the prostate and the rectum. Denonvilliers' fascia is incised, and the posterior rectal plane is dissected widely to the apex of the prostate, leaving the prostate hanging by the pedicles and lateral attachments.

3.4.7. STEP 7: EARLY RETROGRADE ATHERMAL PRESERVATION OF THE NEUROVASCULAR BUNDLES (NVB) (FIG. 7)

If nerve sparing is indicated, it can be performed in an antegrade or retrograde manner. The dissection is begun by visualizing the lateral borders of the prostate. The assistant provides contralateral traction in order to enhance exposure. The lateral prostatic fascia is then incised with cold scissors and the neurovascular bundle is carefully dissected off the prostate in a retrograde manner athermally. By using this technique the NVB is clearly delineated allowing precise placement of Hem-o-lok® clips on the pedicles. Once the apex is reached the NVB can be seen in proximity to the urethra. It must be released from the periurethral tissue using cold scissors to prevent injury during the anastomosis.

3.4.8. STEP 8: APICAL DISSECTION (FIG. 8)

Cold scissors are used to divide the dorsal venous complex and a long urethral stump is developed. The magnification provides excellent visualization, allowing complete dissection of the apex and urethra. Under direct vision, the urethra is incised at the apex of the prostate to release completely.

3.4.9. STEP 9: LYMPH NODE DISSECTION

The lymph node dissection is begun by identifying the landmarks of the pubic ramus and the iliac artery and vein. The lymph node packet is then grasped with the fourth arm, and the scissors and PK dissector are

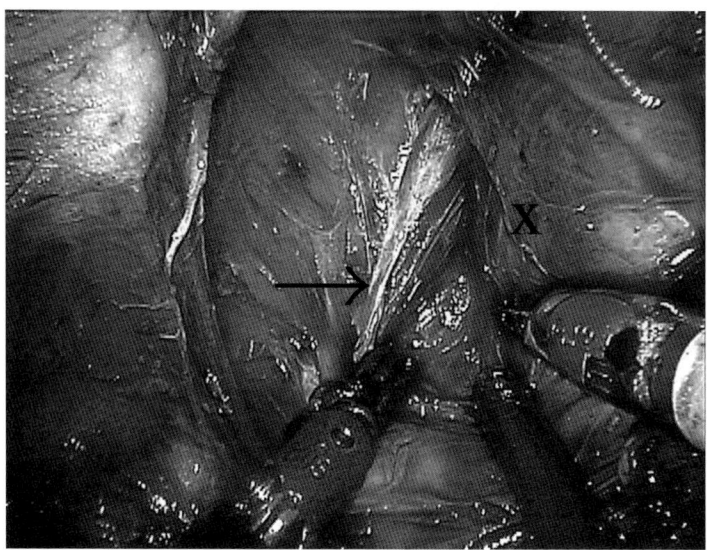

Fig. 7. Neurovascular bundle release. The left neurovascular bundle (*arrow*) is released early with incision of the lateral prostatic fascia and identification of the plane between prostate (*X*) and neurovascular bundle.

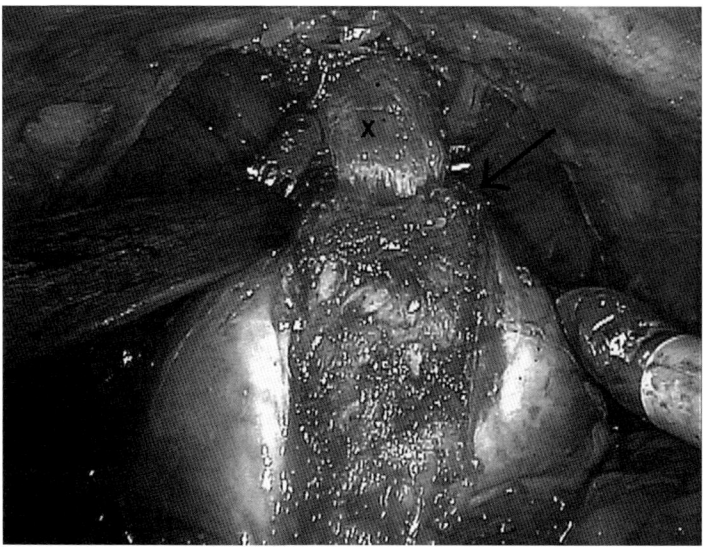

Fig. 8. Apical dissection. The urethra (*X*) is retracted anteriorly to aid in visualization of the prostate apex (*arrow*).

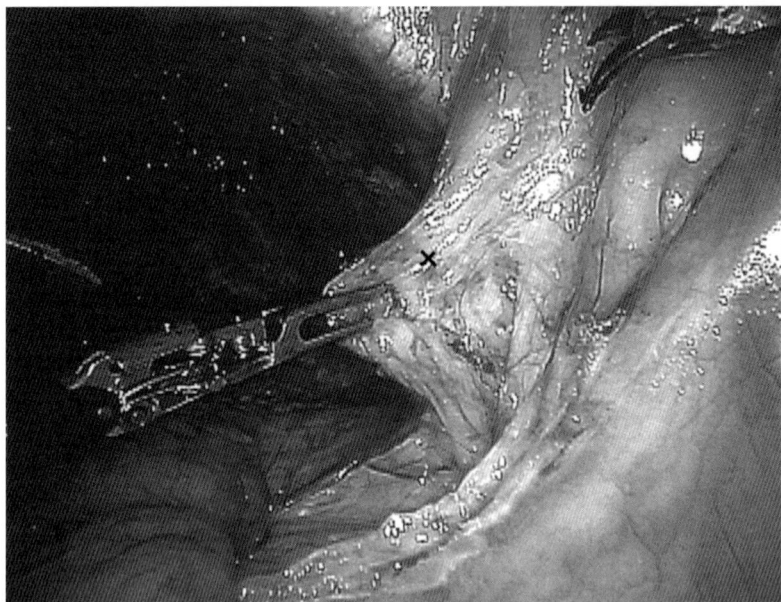

Fig. 9. Lymph node dissection. Lymph node packet (*X*) is grasped with the fourth robotic arm and retracted away from the obturator nerve and iliac vessels.

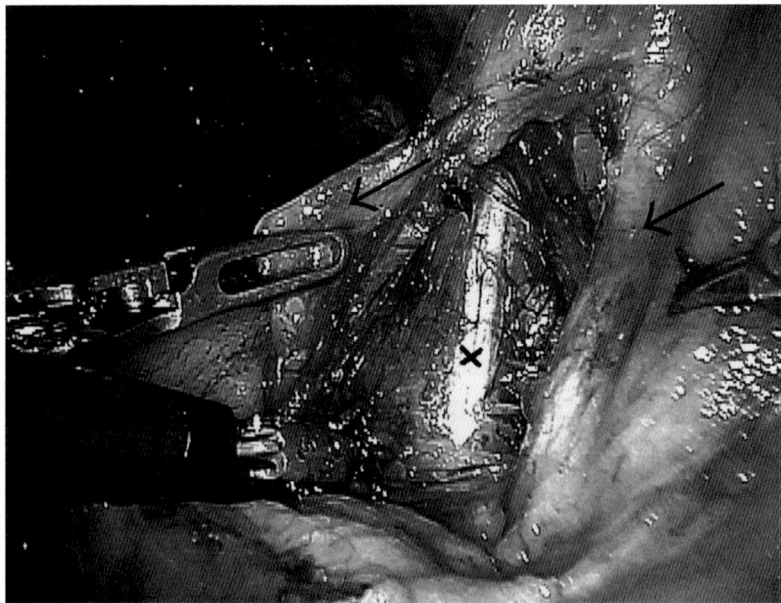

Fig. 10. Identification of obturator nerve during node dissection. Lymph node packet (*small arrow*), iliac vessels (*small arrow*), preserved obturator nerve (*x*).

used to dissect the lymph node packet out of the obturator fossa (Fig. 9) The packet is then swept off the iliac vein to visualize the obturator nerve (Fig. 10) The PK dissector is used to ligate the small feeder vessels taking care to avoid the nerve or the vascular structures running with it.

3.4.10. STEP 10: URETHROVESICAL ANASTOMOSIS

The urethra and bladder are then reapproximated using a continuous stitch of two 3-0 Monocryl sutures (RB1 needle) of different colors that are tied together, with each individual length being 20 cm. Ten knots are placed when tying together the sutures to provide a bolster for the anastomosis. First, the posterior urethral anastomosis is performed with one arm of the suture in a clockwise direction from the 5- to 10-o'clock position. This is followed by completion of the anterior anastomosis with the second arm of the suture in an anticlockwise direction until reaching the 10-o'clock position. Both sutures are tied on the uretrol stump.

4. OUTCOMES

4.1. Operative Time

It is often difficult to compare operative times between various series due to variations in reporting of operative time to include setup, pelvic lymph node dissection, or both. There is an initial learning curve not only for the surgeon with the procedure but also for the operating room staff with setup of the robot. The mean operative time for reported robotic series ranges from 141 to 540 min (Table 1; (1–10,14,16,18–32)). In our experience, our operative time declined from a mean of 202 min for our first 50 cases to 141 min for the last 50 cases in a series of 200 cases (32). Our operative times have now declined further to the range of 90 min as our series has matured and advanced to >1,000 cases.

4.2. Blood Loss and Transfusion

As with any surgery, significant blood loss can occur with any form of prostatectomy. The transfusion rate after RALP has been reported to be 0–16.6% [3-9, 14, 16, 26, 28, 30, 32]. It is known that transfusion rates do not always accurately represent blood loss associated with a procedure. A patient may have significant blood loss and still not require transfusion, which is dependent on surgeon variability with transfusion criteria. Decreased intraoperative blood loss has been reported to be a hallmark advantage of laparoscopic prostatectomy (21,22,33–40). Because most intraoperative blood loss originates

Table 1

Operative Characteristics and Outcomes of RALP

	Mean age (range)	Number of patients	Mean PSA in ng/mL (range)	Access	Number of assistants	Mean operative time in min. (range)	Mean EBL in cc (range)	Transfusion rate (%)	% Positive margins
Abbou et al. (3) (2001)	63 years (NR)	1	7 (NR)	TP	1	420 (NR)	300 (NR)	0	0
Pasticier et al. (4) (2001)	58 years (55–63)	5	12.4 (6–23)	TP	1	222 (150–381)	800 (700–1600)	0	20
Binder et al. (5) (2001)[a]	60.5 years (57–69)	10	6.4 (0.5–22.4)	TP	1	540[a] (325–660)	NR	10	30
Rassweiler et al. (6) (2001)[a]	47 years (40–55)	6	9.7 (2.4–12)	TP	2	315[a] (242–480)	NR	16.6	0
Samadi et al. (28) (2002)	67 years (58–71)	11	8.9 (3.9–32)	TP	1	300 (200–420)	900 (400–1600)	NR	36.4
Menon et al. (16) (2002)	60.7 years (NR)	40	5.7 (NR)	TP	2	274 (NR)	256 (NR)	0	17.5
Menon et al. (8) (2003)	59.9 years (42–76)	200	6.2 (0.6–41)	TP	2	160[a] (71–315)	153 (NR)	0	6
Menon et al. (9) (2003)[a]	NR	100	NR	TP	2	165[a] 135 (NR)	150 (25–525)	NR	4
Bentas et al. (31) (2003)	NR	40	NR	TP	NR	498 (NR)	570 (NR)	NR	NR
Ahlering et al. (14) (2003)	61.4 years (46–71)	45	7.3	TP	1	207	134 (25–350)	0	35.5
Worlfram et al. (30) (2003)	63 years (45–71)	81	8.96 (1.5–40)	TP	1	250 (150–390)	300 (100–1500)	12	22.2
Ahlering et al. (26) (2004)	62.9 years (43–78)	60	8.1 (0.6–62)	TP	1	231 (160–340)	105 (25–400)	0	16.7
Cathelineau et al. (7) (2004)	NR	70 TP 35 EP	8 (4–24)	TP/EP	1	180 (120–190)	500 (150–2000)	6	22
Patel et al. (37) (2005)	59.5(40–78)	200	7.1 (1–90)	TP	1	141.2 (NR)	75 (NR)	0	10.5

[a] includes pelvic lymph node dissection

from the venous sinuses, the tamponade effect created by pnuemoperi-
toneum helps to diminish blood loss *(41)*. In addition, early identification and precise ligation of vessels facilitates the limitation of blood
loss. In many of the RALP series from the United States, there has
been a 0% transfusion rate after RALP *(8,14,16,26,42)*. Menon et al.
(17) report a 0% transfusion rate after 1,100 RALP. In an earlier publi-
cation Tewari et al. *(11)* report a significantly higher rate of transfusion after RRP (67%) compared with RALP (0%) in their single institution series comparing 100 RRPs performed by different surgeons and
200 RALPs performed by a single surgeon. Menon et al. *(16)* have
also reported a higher rate of transfusion after LRP (2.5%) compared
with RALP (0%). The mean estimated blood loss in RALP series is
75–900 cc [Table1; *(3–9,14,16,26,28,30–32)*].

5. FUNCTIONAL OUTCOMES

5.1. Erectile Function

Theoretically, de novo erectile dysfunction after prostatectomy occurs
due to injury of the NVB. Damage to these structures can occur by direct
incision, incorporation of the nerve into hemostatic suture or clips, and
thermal or traction injury. Younger age, better preoperative potency, and
extent of NVB preservation are factors that have been shown to affect
postoperative return of erectile function *(16,43,44)*.

Overall, potency rates after RRP are reported to be 62–68% at high-
volume centers, but they have been reported to be as low as 10–30%
in patient-reported surveys *(44–54)*. In a series by Quinlan et al. *(44)*,
potency rates are 90% for men younger than 50 undergoing RRP, with
preservation of one or both neurovascular bundles with a reduction in
potency rate for men older than 50, especially if both neurovascular
bundles are not preserved. Walsh et al. *(55)* have also reported an overall
rate of potency defined by intercourse with or without the use of sildenafil
to be 38% at 3 months, 54% at 6 months, 73% at 12 months, and 86%
at 18 months.

It has been proposed that RALP may prevent damage to the neurovascular bundle because dissection occurs in an antegrade manner reducing
traction on the nerve and better vision due to magnification and reduced
blood in the surgical field allowing a more precise dissection and
preventing inadvertent incision or incorporation into suture or clip. In their
initial comparative series from a single center, Menon et al. *(16)* reported
a potency rate of 29.4% (5/17) for RALP at mean follow-up of 1.5 months
compared with 25% (3/12) in the LRP group at a mean follow-up of

6.5 months. In their initial series, Ahlering et al. *(14)* only had two preoperatively potent (SHIM >20) patients with adequate follow-up, and they reported a 50% rate of potency at 6–9 months with the postoperatively impotent patient receiving only a unilateral nerve sparing procedure. In a recent series of 565 RALP, Tewari et al. *(11)* report 82% of preoperatively potent patients younger than age 60 had return of some sexual activity and 64% were having sexual intercourse after 6 months. In patients older than 60, 75% had some return of sexual activity and 38% having intercourse at 6 months postoperative. In an earlier series *(11)*, they also compared the outcomes of 200 RALP with those of 100 RRPs performed over the same period, and they reported a more rapid return of erection after RALP (50% return at a median follow-up of 180 days for RALP vs. 440 days for RRP; $p < 0.05$) and a more rapid return to intercourse (50% at 340 days for RALP vs. <50% at >700 days for RRP). Of note, both Menon and Ahlering have noticed improved potency rates after scissors and bipolar electrocautery became available for use with the da Vinci Surgical System (Intuitive Surgical) in the posterior dissection *(8,14)*.

Chien et al. *(56)* recently reported a new clipless technique for nerve preservation. The NVB was dissected in an antegrade manner with point use of bipolar cautery to control vessels. Their results showed return to baseline potency rates of 47, 54, 66, and 69% at 1, 3, 6, and 12 months postprostatectomy.

No consensus exists on the ideal tools to document preoperative and postoperative potency in relation to any form of prostatectomy. There also seems to be great variation in the methodology used for describing potency outcomes amongst all available literature for RRP, LRP, and RALP *(19,34,35,38,57,58)*. However, it does seem that LRP and RALP have similar rates of postoperative potency compared to the best-reported rates after RRP.

5.2. Continence

One of the primary surgical objectives when performing prostatectomy is maintenance of continence. This is often a significant area of concern for the patient when considering treatment options. Precise mucosa-to-mucosa approximation and optimal preparation of the urethral stump are important in preservation of continence and prevention of stricture *(12)*. Younger age, preservation of the neurovascular bundle, and absence of preoperative stricture also have been reported to increase the chance of retaining or regaining continence after surgery *(43)*.

In an earlier series of RRP, the rates of incontinence based on patient-reported surveys was as high as 50% *(46–49)*. Walsh et al. *(55)* reported continence (no pad usage in past 4 weeks) to be 54% at 3 months, 80%

at 6 months, 93% at 12 months, and 93% at 18 months. The pad free rate after RRP at 3 months postoperative has been reported to be between 50 and 76% *(26,59,60)*. The majority of series report continence rates after RRP to be >90% and up to 95% in one series at 12 months postoperatively *(43,51–54,59,61,62)*.

It has been proposed that RALP can potentially result in better continence rates or earlier return of continence by improved preservation of urethral sphincter and urethral length. The theory is that superb visualization of the apex allows the surgeon to gently sweep away urethral sphincter muscular tissue from the anterior prostate and improved hemostasis prevents blood from obscuring the apex leading to inadvertent injury to the sphincter *(41)*. Ahlering et al. *(14)* have reported continence rates of 33, 63, and 81% at 1 week, 1 month, and 3 months after RALP. In a comparative study, Ahlering et al. *(26)* found no significant difference in overall continence rates after RALP (76%) compared with RRP (75%) when performed by the same surgeon. However, Tewari et al. *(11)* have shown return to continence to be quicker in the RALP group with 50% being continent at 44 days compared with 160 days for RRP. In the landmark initial reports of RALP, Pasticier *(4)* reported 80% of patient to be continent at 9 days postoperative, and Binder *(5)* reported a 50% rate of continence at 1 month. Recently, Menon et al. *(12)* have reported a continence rate (no pads) of 96% at 3 months postoperatively. In our study of 200 patients, continence was described as the use of no pads daily, and continence at 1, 3, 6, 9, and 12 months was 47, 82, 89, 92, and 98%, respectively *(32)*.

Return of continence does seem to be earlier for RALP with a trend toward improved overall continence rates (98% for RALP vs. 95% in RRP in best-reported results), even when including cases in the learning curve.

5.3. Oncologic

The primary goal of surgical intervention for prostate cancer is oncologic cure. Men with high tumor stage, large tumor volume, multiple positive biopsies, high biopsy grade, and high preoperative prostate-specific antigen (PSA) are more likely to have a positive margin after surgery *(63–65)*. Positive margin is a well-established independent risk factor for PSA recurrence *(42)*. As such, any modifications of the gold standard must provide for equivalent oncologic outcomes to be considered viable options of treatment. It is theorized that the lack of tactile feedback associated with LRP and RALP may prevent equivalent oncologic results because the surgeon is unable to palpate the tumor. Others have theorized that magnified three-dimensional vision and minimal blood in the surgical field can improve vision helping the dissection and potentially lead to decreased positive surgical margins.

Most contemporary open RRP series report overall positive margin rates (PMRs) of 12–25% *(62,65)*. In a literature review, Weider and Soloway *(64)* reported positive margin rates after RRP to range from 0 to 77%, with an overall average of 28% in reviewed RRP series. In this review, they also report PMRs for T2a disease to be 0–38%, with an average of 17%; 11–77%, with an average of 36% for T2b; and 25–59%, with an average of 53% for T3 disease *(64)*. Eastham et al. *(63)* report significantly increased risk of positive margins with RRP when performed by surgeons with lower surgical volume.

In RALP, the surgeon is made devoid of tactile feedback as laparoscopic instruments are controlled by robotic arms without haptic feedback. With this, the fear of poorer oncologic outcomes were heightened initially, but it has subsided as most surgeons can overcome the lack of tactile feedback due to the improved three-dimensional vision and magnification. The reported PMRs after RALP in reported series ranges from 0 to 36.4% *(3–9,14,16,26,28,30–32)*. When broken down by stage, PMRs ranges from 0 to 16.7% for T2a, 0–33.3% for T2b, 0–20% for T2, 0–81.8% for T3a, 20–50% for T3b, 0–75% for combined T3, and 33.3–66.6% for T4 (Table 2; 3–9, 14, 16, 26, 28, 30–32]). This seems to be similar to those outcomes for RRP. In a comparative single-surgeon series, Ahlering et al. *(26)* reported a trend toward higher rate of positive surgical margins in open RRP group (20%) compared with the RALP group (16.7%), even though it did not reach statistical significance due to low sample size. In this same series, they reported PMRs associated with T2 disease of 4.5% for RALP compared with 9.1% in RRP *(26)*. In our series of 500 the PMR was 9.4% for the entire series. The positive margin rate for cases 1–100 was 13%, 8% (101–200), 13% (201–300), 5% (301–400), and 8% (401–500). PMR was 2% for T2a tumors, 4% for T2b, 2.5% for T2c, 24% for T3a, 40% for T3b, and 63% for T4a. For organ-confined disease (T2), the margin rate was 2.5% and 31% for non organ-confined disease. There were a total of 47 positive margins, 26 (56%) posterolateral, 4 (8.5%) apical, 4 (8.5%) bladder neck, 2 (4%) seminal vesicle, and 11 (23%) multifocally.

True oncologic outcome can only be evaluated based on long- term survival and recurence data. Since LRP and RALP are so new, this data is not available at this time. Short term PSA data from the majority of series is promising. The variability in margin status reporting and pathologic specimen handling also makes cross series analysis very difficult. This

Table 2
Positive Margin Rates

	Number of patients	PT_1	PT_{2a}	PT_{2b}	PT_2	PT_{3a}	PT_{3b}	PT_{3a+b}	PT_4	PT_{3+4}
Abbou et al. (3) (2001)	1	—	—	—	—	0/1 (0%)	—	0/1 (0%)	—	0/1 (0%)
Pasticier et al. (4) (2001)	5	—	0/2 (0%)	1/3 (33.3%)	1/5 (20%)	—	—	—	—	—
Binder et al. (5) (2001)	10	—	0/2 (0%)	0/4 (0%)	0/6 (0%)	2/2 (100%)	1/2 (50%)	3/4 (75%)	—	3/4 (75%)
Rassweiler et al. (6) (2001)	6	—	0/3 (0%)	0/2 (0%)	0/5 (0%)	0/1 (0%)	NR	NR	—	0/1 (0%)
Samadi et al. (3) (2002)	11	—	NR	NR	1/8 (12.5%)	NR	NR	2/3 (66.6%)	—	2/3 (66.6%)
Ahlering et al. (14) (2003)	45	—	1/6 (16.7%)	3/21 (14.3%)	4/27 (14.8%)	9/11 (81.8%)	1/5 (20%)	10/16 (62.5%)	2/3 (66.7%)	12/19 (63.2%)
Wolfram et al. (30) (2003)	81	—	NR	NR	7/55 (12.7%)	NR	NR	11/26 (42.3%)	—	11/26 (42.3%)
Ahlering et al. (26) (2004)	60	—	NR	NR	2/44 (4.5%)	NR	NR	NR	NR	8/16 (50%)
Cathelineau et al. (7) (2004)	105	—	NR	NR	9/75 (11.7%)	NR	NR	13/30 (43%)	—	13/30 (43%)

prevents definitive comparison of RALP, RPP, and LRP in regards to superiority of oncologic outcome.

6. CONCLUSIONS

Transperitoneal robotic assisted laparoscopic radical prostatectomy is a promising procedure in evolution. It is estimated that in 2007, approximately 60% of all prostatectomies will be performed robotically.

The limitations of robotic technology such as bulky instrumentation and lack of haptic feedback seem to be outweighed by the advantages of improved visualization and miniature wristed instrumentation.

Short-term data is growing quickly, and is encouraging compared with the current gold standard in terms of functional and oncologic outcomes. As robotic technology evolves and becomes more prevalent, we expect to see continued adoption, innovation, and improved surgical outcomes.

REFERENCES

1. Jemal A, Tiwari R, Murray T, Ghafoor A, Samuels A (2004) Cancer statistics–2004. CA Cancer J Clin 54:8.
2. Holmberg L, Bill-Axelson A, Helgesen F et al (2002) A randomized trial comparing radical prostatectomy with watchful waiting in early prostate cancer. N Eng J Med 347:781.
3. Abbou C-C, Hoznek A, Salomon L et al (2001) Laparoscopic radical prostatectomy with a remote controlled robot. J Urol 165:1964.
4. Pasticier G, Rietbergen JBW, Guillonneau B, Fromont G, Menon M, Vallancien G (2001) Robotically assisted laparoscopic radical prostatectomy: feasibility study in men. Eur Urol 40:70.
5. Binder J, Kramer W (2001) Robotically-assisted laparoscopic radical prostatectomy. BJU Int 87:408.
6. Rassweiler J, Frede T, Seemann O, Stock C, Sentker L (2001) Telesurgical laparoscopic radical prostatectomy. Eur Urol 40:75.
7. Cathelineau X, Rozet F, Vallancien G (2004) Robotic radical prostatectomy: the European experience. Urol Clin N Am 31:693.
8. Menon M et al (2003) Robotic radical prostatectomy and the Vattikuti Urology Institute technique: an interim analysis of results and technical points. Urology 61 (Suppl 4A):10.
9. Menon M, Tewari A, Peabody J et al (2003) Vattikutti Institute prostatectomy: Technique. J Urol 169:2289.
10. Menon M, Tewari A, Baise, Guillonneau B, Vallancien G (2002) Prospective comparison of radical retropubic prostatectomy and robot-assisted anatomic prostatectomy: The Vattikutti Urology Institute experience. Urology 60: 864.
11. Tewari A, Srivasatava A, Menon M et al (2003) A prospective comparison of radical retropubic and robot-assisted prostatectomy: experience in one institution. BJU Int 92:205.

12. Menon M. Hemal AK, Tewari A, Shrivastava A, Bhandari A (2004) The technique of apical dissection of the prostate and urethrovesical anastomosis in robotic radical prostatectomy. BJU Int 93:715.
13. Hemal AK, Menon M (2004) Robotics in urology. Curr Opin Urol 12:89.
14. Ahlering TE, Skarecky D, Lee D, Clayman RV (2003) Successful transfer of open surgical skills to a laparoscopic environment using a robotic interface: initial experience with laparoscopic radical prostatectomy. J Urol 170:1738.
15. Bhandari A, Peabody JO, Tiwari A et al (2004) Does surgical robot assist in safe learning of laparoscopic radical prostatectomy? AUA Abstract.
16. Menon M, Shrivastava A, Tewari et al (2002) Laparoscopic and robot assisted radical prostatectomy: establishment of a structured program and preliminary analysis of outcome. J Urol 168:945.
17. Menon M, Tewari A, Peabody JO et al (2004) Vattikuti Institute prostatectomy, a technique of robotic radical prostatectomy for management of localized carcinoma of the prostate: experience of over 1100 cases. Urol Clin N Am 31:701.
18. Scheusler WW, Schlaum PG, Clayman RV, Kavousi LR (1997) Laparoscopic radical prostatectomy: initial short term experience. Urology 50:854.
19. Guillonneau B, Vallancien G (2000) Laparoscopic radical prostatectomy: the Montsouris experience. J Urol 163:418.
20. Rassweiler J, Seemann O, Schulze M et al (2003) Laparoscopic versus open radical prostatectomy: comparative study at a single institution. J Urol 169:1689.
21. Rassweiler J, Sentker L, Seeman O, Hatzinger, Rumpelt HJ (2001) Laparoscopic radical prostatectomy with the Heilbronn technique: an analysis of the first 180 cases. J Urol 166:2010.
22. Turk I, Deger S, Winkelmann B, Schonberger B, Loening S (2001) Laparoscopic radical prostatectomy. Eur Urol 40:46.
23. Salomon L. Levrel O, Taille A, Anastasiadis AG, Abbou CC (2002) Radical prostatectomy by the retropubic, perineal, and laparoscopic approach: 12 years of experience in one center. Eur Urol 42:104.
24. Eden CG, Chaill D, Vass JA, Adams TH, Dauleh MI (2002) Laparoscopic radical prostatectomy: the initial UK series. BJU 90:876.
25. Sulser T, Guillonneau B, Vallancien G et al (2001) Complication and initial experience with 1228 laparoscopic radical prostatectomies at 6 European centers. J Urol 165 (Suppl):150.
26. Ahlering TE, Woo D, Eichel L et al (2004) Robot-assisted versus open radical prostatectomy: a comparison of one surgeon's outcomes. Urology 63:820.
27. Abbou CC, Hoznek A, Olsson LE et al (2002) Telerobotic laparoscopic radical prostatectomy. AUA Abstract.
28. Samadi DB, Nadu A, Olsson E et al (2002) Robot assisted laparoscopic radical prostatectomy: Initial experience in eleven patients. AUA Abstract.
29. Fumo M, Shrivastava A, DePeralta M et al (2003) Does routine preservation of the neurovascular bundle result in poor oncological outcomes in patients undergoing robotic radical prostatectomy? AUA Abstract.
30. Wolfram M, Brautigam R, Engl T et al (2003) Robotic-assisted laparoscopic radical prostatectomy: the Frankfurt technique. World J Urol 21:128.
31. Bentas W, Wolfram M, Jones J et al (2003) Robotic technology and the translation of open radical prostatectomy to laparoscopy: the early Frankfurt experience with robotic radical prostatectomy and one year follow up. Eur Urol 44:175.
32. Patel VR, Tully AS, Linday J (2005) Robotic radical prostatectomy in the community setting: the learning curve and beyond: initial 200 cases. J Urol 174:269.

33. Guillonneau B, Rozet F, Barrett E, Cathelineau X, Vallancien G (2001) Laparo-scopic radical prostatectomy: assessment after 240 procedures. Urol Clin N Am 28:189.
34. Guillonneau B, el-Fettouh H, Baumert H et al (2003) Laparoscopic radical prosta-tectomy: oncological evaluation after 1,000 cases at Montsouris Institute. J Urol 169:1261.
35. Hoznek A, Salomon L, Olsson LE et al (2001) Laparoscopic radical prostatectomy: the Creteil experience. Eur Urol 40:38.
36. Gill IS, Zippe CD (2001) Laparoscopic radical prostatectomy: technique. Urol Clin North Am 28:423.
37. Dahl D, L'esperance JO, Trainer AF et al (2001) Laparoscopic radical prostate-ctomy: initial 70 cases at a U.S. university medical center. Urology 58:570.
38. Turk I, Deger S, Winkelmann B et al (2001) Laparoscopic radical prostatectomy: technical aspects and experience with 125 cases. Eur Urol 40:46.
39. Anastasiadis AG, Salomon L, Katz R et al (2003) Radical retropubic versus laparo-scopic prostatectomy: A prospective comparison of functional outcome. Urology 62:292.
40. Fabrizio MD, Tuerk I, Schellhammer PF (2003) Laparoscopic radical prostate-ctomy: decreasing the learning curve using a mentor initiated approach. J Urol 169:2063.
41. Smith JA Jr (2004) Robotically assisted laparoscopic prostatectomy: an assessment of its contemporary role in the surgical management of localized prostate cancer. Am J Surg 188:63S.
42. Ahlering TE, Eichel L, Edwards RA, Lee DI, Skarecky DW (2004) Robotic radical prostatectomy: a technique to reduce pT2 positive margins. Urology 64:1224.
43. Eastham J, Scardino P (2002) Radical prostatectomy. In: Campbell's urology, 4th edn. W. B. Saunders, Philadelphia, PA, p 3080.
44. Quinlan DM, Epstein GI, Carter BS, Walsh PC (1991) Sexual function following radical prostatectomy: influence of preservation of neurovascular bundles. J Urol 145:998.
45. Catalona WJ, Carvalhal GF, Mager DE, Smith DS (1999) Potency, continence, and complication rates in 1870 Consecutive radical retropubic prostatectomies. J Urol 162:433.
46. Fowler FJ Jr, Barry MJ, Lu-Yao G et al (1993) Patient-reported complications and follow up treatment after radical prostatectomy. Urology 42:622.
47. Geary ES, Dendinger TE, Frieha FS et al (1995) Nerve sparing radical prostate-ctomy: a different view. J Urol 154:145.
48. Geary ES, Dendinger TE, Frieha FS et al (1995) Incontinence and vesical neck strictures following radical retropubic prostatectomy. Urology 45:1000.
49. Talcott JA, Ricker P, Propert KJ et al (1997) Patient reported impotence and incontinence after nerve sparing radical prostatectomy. J Natl Cancer Inst 89:1117.
50. Moul JW, Mooneyhan RN, Kao TC et al (1998) Preoperative and operative factors to predict incontinence, impotence, and stricture after radical prostatectomy. Prostate Cancer Prostatic Dis 5: 242.
51. Walsh PC, Partin AW, Epstein JI (1994) Cancer control and quality of life following anatomical radical retropubic prostatectomy: results at 10 years. J Urol 152:1831.
52. Catalona WJ, Basler JW (1993) Return of erections and urinary continence following nerve sparing radical retropubic prostatectomy. J Urol 150: 905.
53. Eastham JA, Kattan MW, Roger SE et al (1996) Risk factors for urinary inconti-nence after radical prostatectomy. J Urol 156:1707.

54. Palapattu JS, Stapelton AM, Seale-Hawkins CK et al (1996) A change in technique in radical retropubic prostatectomy markedly improves post-operative potency. J Urol 155:647a.

55. Walsh PA, Marschke P, Ricker D, Burnett AI (2000) Patient-reported urinary continence and sexual function after anatomic radical prostatectomy. Urology 55:58.

56. Chien GW, Mikhail AA, Orvieto MA et al (2005) Modified clipless antegrade nerve preservation in robotic-assisted laparoscopic radical prostatectomy with validated sexual function evaluation. Urology 66:419.

57. Rassweiler J, Sentker L, Seemann O et al (2000) Laparoscopic radical prostatectomy: technique and first experiences. Akt Urol 31:238.

58. Bollens R, Vanden Bossche M, Roumeguere T et al (2001) Extraperitoneal laparoscopic radical prostatectomy: results after 50 cases. Eur Urol 40:65.

59. Walsh PC (2000) Patient-reported urinary continence and sexual function after anatomic radical prostatectomy. J Urol 164:242.

60. Lepor H, Nieder AM, Fraiman MC (2001) Early removal of urinary catheter after radical retropubic prostatectomy is both feasible and desirable. Urology 58:425.

61. Lepor H, Nieder AM, Ferrandino MN (2001) Intraoperative and postoperative complications of radical retropubic prostatectomies in a consecutive series of 1,000 cases. J Urol 166:1729.

62. Zincke H, Bergstralh Ej, Blute ML et al (1994) Radical prostatectomy for clinically localized prostate cancer: long-term results of 1,143 patients from a single institution. J Clin Oncol 12:2254–2263.

63. Eastham JA, Kattan MW, Riedel E et al (2003) Variations among individual surgeons in the rate of positive surgical margins in radical prostatectomy specimens. J Urol 170:2292.

64. Weider JA, Soloway MS (1998) Incidence, etiology, location, prevention and treatment of positive surgical margins after radical prostatectomy for prostate cancer. J Urol 160:299.

65. Hull GW, Rabbani F, Abbas F, Wheeler TM, Kattan MW, Scardino PT (2002) Cancer control with radical prostatectomy alone in 1,000 consecutive patients. J Urol 167:528.

5 Extraperitoneal Robotic Radical Prostatectomy

Michael P. Esposito, Vincent J. Lanteri, and Gregory Lovallo

1. INTRODUCTION

Although methodologic variations among studies complicate precise attempts at comparison *(1)*, over the past 8 years in the United States and Europe, minimally invasive laparoscopic radical prostatectomy has proved to be a safe and effective alternative to traditional open radical retropubic prostatectomy that has significantly reduced its morbidity. Many studies have demonstrated a considerable decrease in recovery time, blood loss, transfusion rates, and hospital stay. In addition, a reduction in time to full urinary continence, return of potency, and pathologic surgical positive margin rates has been reported by several groups *(2)*.

Robotically assisted surgical systems have been increasingly used in complex laparoscopic procedures encompassing the general, pediatric, cardiac, gynecologic, and urologic surgical disciplines *(3–8)*. Robotically assisted laparoscopic radical prostatectomy (rLRP) was first performed in Germany *(9,10)* and France *(11)* by using past laparoscopic experience as a guide. Armed with sophisticated and innovative robotic technology, practitioners were able to improve operative times and surgical results. Furthermore, the sophisticated technology has enabled urologic surgeons trained only in the traditional procedure to perform this complex operation with a considerably shorter learning curve *(12–16)*.

Early reports demonstrated the efficacy and safety of the robotic technique. When the technology was Food and Drug Administration-approved for use in the United States in 2001, surgeons in several centers chose to convert from pure laparoscopic procedures to using robotic assistance to perform minimally invasive prostatectomy *(17–21)*.

From: *Current Clinical Urology: Urologic Robotic Surgery*
Edited by: J. A. Stock, M. P. Esposito, and V. J. Lanteri © Humana Press, Totowa, NJ

The initial set of needle drivers and monopolar hook cautery instruments has since been expanded to include others specifically designed for use during the careful atraumatic steps of a radical prostatectomy. These range from the bipolar dissector, bipolar Maryland dissector, ultrasonic scalpel, and monopolar curved scissors to retracting instruments such as the ProGrasp and Cobra graspers that have extra grip and tissue grasping capability. Robotic surgery has given rise to modifications in techniques used in nerve sparing (22–24) and nerve grafting (25); pedicle litigation (26); apical dissection (27,28); and setup of the patient, ports, and robotic system (29–31).

As the text throughout this book testifies, although the four-arm da Vinci Surgical System (Intuitive Surgical, Sunnyvale, CA) is well suited to and advantageous for many urological surgical procedures, it is ideal for allowing access to hard-to-reach anatomy deep in the pelvis for ablative prostate surgery (32).

The extraperitoneal approach to rLRP (33) closely resembles the approach to Walsh's anatomic radical prostatectomy. By creating an anatomic barrier to the contents of the peritoneal cavity, the extraperitoneal space (1) allows for a more familiar working space and anatomy for most contemporary urologic surgeons; (2) permits significantly less Trendelenberg positioning (15 versus 35°); (3) potentially contains both anastomotic urine leaks, thereby preventing urinary ascites, and periprostatic hemorrhage, potentially precluding the need for surgical exploration; and (4) seems to allow more comfortable recovery through lower incidence of painful ileus (34,35).

2. PREOPERATIVE ASSESSMENT

The preoperative evaluation of any patient being considered for surgical treatment of prostate cancer should be comprehensive. The same is true when a patient is being considered for rLRP. Surgeons with less experience are advised during the initial learning curve to choose patients with no history of prior abdominal surgery, a body mass index <30, and prostate volume <50 cc (36).

The patient's past surgical history must be thorough and complete, because previous operations may preclude surgical treatment, or at a minimum, prompt a change in approach from transperitoneal to extraperitoneal or vice versa. The first 50 cases should exclude patients with histories of prior prostatic surgery. Due to the likelihood of intestinal adhesions, a history of prior abdominal surgery dictates caution during access and exposure of the prostate. In cases of either inguinal, umbilical, or incisional hernia surgery, operative reports should be reviewed to assess for the use of mesh material that can result in dense adhesions.

Possible cardiovascular disease may require investigation with stress testing or cardiac catheterization, and like past history, makes it prudent to obtain cardiac clearance. A history of lung disease or smoking may require pulmonary function testing and preoperative optimization with bronchodilators. Physical conditioning, weight loss, and cessation of smoking also may improve recovery.

Proper clinical staging with bone scan and computed tomography in selected patients is indicated. Endorectal coil magnetic resonance imaging of the prostate with or without spectroscopy should be considered in selected patients as well. An evaluation of presurgical potency with a validated questionnaire should be performed. A realistic assessment of oncologic outcomes based on available personal experience data and nomograms *(37–39)* should be discussed with the patient and loved ones.

We perform flexible cystoscopy on all patients being considered for robotic radical prostatectomy to assess for urethral stricture, aberrant prostatic anatomy, and location of ureteral orifices in relation to the prostatic lobes. A thorough evaluation of voiding history that determines level of storage and emptying voiding symptoms, and a history of incontinence and type, if present, are extremely important. This information may necessitate further evaluation with urodynamic studies and additional counseling concerning postoperative voiding expectations. Patients should be given instructions for preoperative Kegel exercises, and a schedule for these exercises should be planned.

3. ANESTHETIC CONSIDERATIONS

We recommend reviewing each patient with the anesthesiologist before beginning the operation. Preparation should include the insertion of an orogastric tube to decompress the stomach and empty the gastric contents. Antibiotic prophylaxis and specific subacute bacterial endocarditis prophylaxis also should also be given if clinically indicated. Because evaluation of urine output as an indication of hydration status is not possible during most of the procedure, the anesthesiologist should hydrate the patient as required for the length of time the patient has been fluid intake restricted and also monitor the blood loss during the procedure and hemodynamic parameters including blood pressure, heart rate, central venous pressure, if available, and insensible losses. Although intravenous fluid replacement (IVF) is of utmost importance, we request, if clinical parameters allow, that the IVF be limited to 1–1.5 liters of i.v. crystalloid until the urethrovesical anastomosis is begun. This practice changes with each patient, especially for replacement in case of increase in either blood loss or procedure length or for start times later in the day. We request that nitrous oxide not be used as an anesthetic agent during the procedure because we have found this to cause bowel distension. Each patient should have packed red blood cells available from either the blood bank or autologous/directed donation.

4. PATIENT POSITIONING

A folded sheet is placed under the supine patient from the axillae to mid-hand level. This sheet is laid over a 0.75-in. 3-ft square gel pad that serves two functions: (1) because we allow the gel pad to contact the patient's shoulders, its tactile properties secure the patient to the table; and (2) the pad cushions the patient. The arms are surrounded with foam pads, and the sheet is used to tuck them to the sides in the anatomic position to protect the ulnar nerve and bony prominences (Fig. 1).

The lower extremities are well padded in boot stirrups that provide full support with weight bearing on padded heels. The lateral proximal fibula must be well padded to protect the peroneal nerve. The legs are spread adequately to allow access to the rectum for bougie manipulation and for

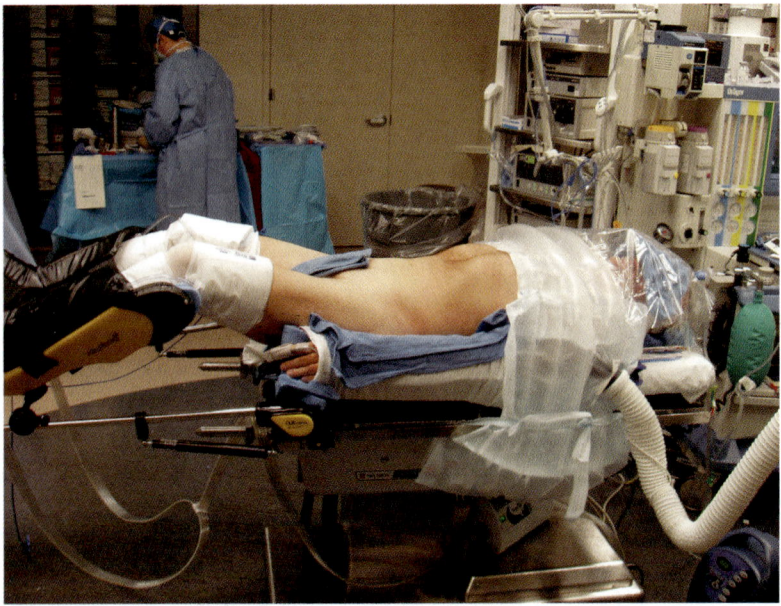

Fig. 1. Patient fully positioned for surgery. Note arms tucked and padded, lower extremities in boot stirrups peroneal nerve padded and protected weight is placed on heels, minimal hip and knee flexion.

positioning of the central column of the robotic cart during the docking process. The legs should be neither internally or externally rotated, but rather they should be kept neutral.

5. EXTRAPERITONEAL ACCESS

Before starting the access procedure, a Foley catheter must always be inserted to decompress the bladder. A left- or right-sided 12-mm curvilinear periumbilical incision is made. Either 2-S or infant Deaver retractors are used during this exposure step. This incision is carried through Campers and Scarpas fascial layers to the surface of the rectus sheath, which is incised with a scalpel just immediately lateral to the linear alba. The sheath is then spread with Metzenbaum scissors to expose the rectus muscle fibers, which are then spread to expose the posterior sheath. The surgeon must be careful to remain above and not pierce the posterior rectus sheath to maintain the proper plane.

Gentle finger dissection is used to make space for a PDB 52 oval-preperitoneal balloon cannula to be placed under the rectus muscle but always above the posterior sheath. The balloon cannula is lubricated and inserted with a twisting motion to contact the superior surface of the pubic symphysis, then directed slightly posterior to it. A 0° 10-mm laparoscope is then inserted, and dilatation is carried out under direct vision. Once the balloon is pumped and starts to inflate and dilate the space, gentle external pressure is used as needed to guide the balloon across the midline. Generally this dilatation requires 28–30 compressions. In case of failure to cross the midline (which is unusual), unilateral ports are inserted, the space is insufflated, and the contralateral space is created using a combination of blunt and sharp dissection. (A long clear trocar such as a 12-mm trocar with a beveled tip is helpful during this step.)

6. TROCAR INSERTION

The balloon device is fully deflated, removed, and replaced with a 12-mm long trocar. Once again, S-type retractors are used to guide the trocar into the proper space, and the extraperitoneal space is insufflated to 15 mmHg CO_2 pressure. A 0 or 30° down telescope is used depending on the preference of the surgeon; the telescope is warmed, and antifog treatment is applied. Carbon dioxide is insufflated through the camera trocar and warmed with a CO_2 gas-warming device.

Once insufflated, the space is inspected locating the bladder inferiorly, the epigastric vessels superomedially, the pubic symphysis caudally, and the peritoneal envelope superolaterally. At times, a layer of transversalis fascia can make it difficult to discern the pubic symphysis, but it will appear more clearly once dissection begins along the surface of the bladder.

Using the tip of the long 12-mm trocar and a 0° telescope, the surgeon creates a space lateral to the epigastric vessels by sweeping the fat and peritoneal envelope cephalad and lateral until tranversus muscle fibers are visible. This step must be performed very carefully, because it is possible to create a peritoneal perforation, which will cause the space to collapse. A 21-gauge finder needle is then used to evaluate whether this space will accommodate the proper placement of an 8-mm robotic trocar. The proper location externally is approximately two fingerbreadths superomedial to the anterior superior iliac spine, an area that usually corresponds to the transversus muscle fibers internally. Once these two areas are located, the 8-mm robotic trocars are placed bilaterally.

7. SALVAGE OF EXTRAPERITONEAL SPACE

Occasionally, the extraperitoneal space is lost due to inadvertent peritoneal insufflation that causes it to collapse. The collapse may result from an obvious peritoneal membrane tear, a thinning of the membrane with no apparent breach, or no discernible cause.

When the extraperitoneal space has collapsed, we have been able to re-expand it by decompressing the peritoneum. At this point, the peritoneal cavity is typically insufflated, and inserting a 5-mm visible entry trocar provides safe entry into the peritoneal cavity for decompression. We have found the Veress needle to be inadequate for this purpose. This trocar allows for either continuous or intermittent venting of the peritoneum.

If the extraperitoneal space cannot be reinsufflated to create adequate space to accommodate trocar insertion or allow adequate maneuvering, the surgeon must decide either to proceed or to convert to a transperitoneal approach. Having found that proceeding with less than optimal space is a struggle, we choose the latter option. Conversion to a transperitoneal approach requires the peritoneal cavity to be directly insufflated via the newly inserted 5-mm ventilation trocar. The 12-mm periumbilical camera trocar is removed and reinserted to traverse the peritoneal membrane, which had originally been avoided. Use of two small retractors helps to identify the peritoneum. The four additional trocars must then be repositioned so that they, too, traverse the peritoneum for clear access to the pelvic anatomy.

Once this process is complete, the patient must be placed in the 35° Trendelenberg position. The procedure is then begun by incising the peritoneum horizontally, because the bladder attachments will already have been lysed.

8. POSITIONING OF THE TROCARS AND ROBOTIC ARMS TO CONTINUE THE EXTRAPERITONEAL PROCEDURE

If an assistant is to be on the left side of the patient, two 8-mm robotic trocars are inserted in the right lower quadrant and one 8-mm trocar in the left lower lateral quadrant. There is only one assistant trocar; we typically insert a bladeless 10-mm trocar or a 10-mm U.S. Surgical VersaStep trocar. These types of trocars are used to increase safety in the area of the epigastric vessels and to preclude the need to close the port site fascia. If trauma occurs and bleeding begins from the epigastric vessels, a laparoscopic fascial closure device may be used to ligate the bleeding vessel.

To avoid external collision, the trocars must be at least 8–10 cm (four fingerbreadths) from one another. The da Vinci S System may be advantageous during the extraperitoneal approach because occasionally the trocars are necessarily somewhat closer together, and the telescoping ability of the robotic arms, allowing a lower profile external component, may preclude external collision. The space around the 12-mm telescopic trocar is closed with a U-stitch so that no air leak occurs. A rectal bougie

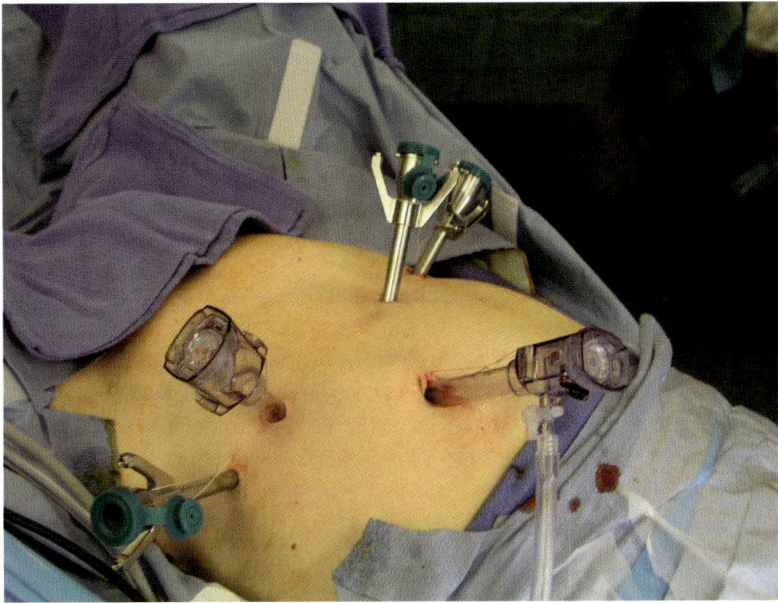

Fig. 2. Configuration of trocars for extraperitoneal case. Two robotic trocars in right lower quadrant, note assistant trocar 12 mm and placed medial to robotic trocar to facilitate assistance deep in the pelvis along left pelvic wall. Telescopic trocar 12 mm and left periumbilical to allow for more operative space for two right sided robotic arms.

EEA size 26 is inserted, and the table placed in the 15° Trendelenberg position (Fig. 2).

In docking the robotic system, the surgeon confirms that there is no contact with the patient or external collision of the robotic arms and that all arms are freely movable in the trajectory of the deep pelvis. If the assistant trocar does not have freely mobile access to the deep pelvis, adjustments can be made by clutching the arms and displacing them away from that instrument.

9. PELVIC SPACE CLEANING

Coagulation settings are bipolar 60-low and monopolar 30 pure cutting-60 medium/coagulation. These settings allow sufficient fulguration of all potential bleeding fat and vessels to keep the procedure bloodless as long as possible. To move through the area, the surgeon views or gently makes contact with the bone of the pubic ramus as a guide.

10. ENDOPELVIC FASCIA OPENING

Depending upon where countertraction is required, the surgeon uses the fourth arm to retract the bladder down, right, or left. After finding and cleaning the endopelvic fascia from apex to bladder level, the surgeon then uses the fourth arm to retract the prostate to one side; by releasing the fascia at the proper reflection from the pelvic wall muscle, this action shows an avascular area that is safe to open. Avoiding the apex for the present, the surgeon opens this area with monopolar shears.

After the endopelvic fascia has been opened from the apex to the bladder level, the apical dissection is performed carefully. If the dorsal vein is inadvertently entered, brisk bleeding may occur. Difficult to control, this bleeding may require temporary increase of the pneumoperitoneum to 18 mmHg or the application of a closure suture.

The lateral areas of the prostate apex have muscle fiber attachments that must be preserved. The dissection is best undertaken with shears and bipolar current. These fibers are released from the superior surface downward by carefully entering the correct plane. These sphincteric fibers should be displaced only enough to allow visualization of the proper area to ligate the dorsal vein. Almost invariably, there are perforating venous channels within these fibers that require coagulation. The dissection should be carried toward the level of the urethra and neurovascular bundle by using minimal to no cautery at this level as to avoid injury of the neurovascular bundle at this location.

The dorsal vein may be cleaned as well by lysing the puboprostatic ligaments and sweeping away the thin layer of muscle from the lateral aspect of the venous complex. The surgeon then ligates the exposed dorsal venous complex. Between the deep part of the venous complex and the anterior surface of the urethra, a subtle step-off is visible. This is the proper plane to pass the ligating suture using 2-0 Vicryl on a CT-1 needle. This suture is placed backhand in a horizontal plane. An additional bunching suture is placed slightly distal to the suspected area of the prostatovesical junction. The Foley catheter can be inflated to 20 cc, and gentle traction can be used to guide placement of this suture at the proper site or on e can squeeze the prostate from both side at the junction to delineate this site. This suture is important because it sets up the transection site to progress in an anatomic manner.

11. LOCALIZATION AND OPENING OF BLADDER NECK

The fat over the prostate is cleaned to the proposed area of the prostatovesical junction, where it is typically adhering. After inflating the Foley catheter balloon to 20 ml, the surgeon places gentle traction on the catheter to delineate the junction. The fourth arm is used to retract the bladder, and the superficial venous channels are well coagulated. The lateral curve of the prostate helps in choosing the proper plane of initial transection.

The superficial veins are then cauterized. Before the bladder neck is entered, a gentle pull on the Foley catheter is used as a guide to the proper junction between the bladder and prostate. By carefully dissecting the bladder from the prostate in a somewhat lateral-to-medial manner, it is possible to locate the area of the prostatic urethra. Once this tapered urethra is cleared, it is followed slightly into the prostate, where the anterior urethra is then opened. Maintaining a small bladder neck will facilitate the urethrovesical anastomosis, and it also may improve continence.

Once the bladder neck is opened anteriorly and laterally, the Foley catheter balloon is deflated. The fourth arm is used to retract the Foley catheter upward; clamping the Foley catheter over a lap pad externally affords internal countertraction. The surgeon then visually confirms the location of the ureteric orifices.

12. POSTERIOR BLADDER NECK TRANSECTION

Posterior bladder neck transection is one of the more difficult steps of the operation. A slight color change between the bladder epithelium and the richer red epithelium overlying the prostate usually signals the correct plane to open. The posterior bladder neck must be completely transected. It is vital to perform this dissection symmetrically and in the correct trajectory to avoid both undermining the trigone and entering the prostate. The correct depth may be inferred from an estimate of the posterior bladder thickness made by gently applying pressure with an instrument directed caudally at the apparent junction of the prostate and posterior bladder neck. During this dissection, the forth-arm is used to lift the posterior part of the prostate. Once the bladder wall is traversed, fatty loose connective tissue covering the seminal vesicles will appear.

This dissection should be carried out slowly because, if the wrong plane is entered, the misdirection may be identified and corrected before too much dissection is carried out. Entrance in the wrong plane is usually heralded by excess bleeding from the bladder or prostate tissue. Reorientation is necessary using the lateral edges and contour of the prostate to guide the dissection. Careful slow dissection will usually salvage the correct plane. It is possible to enter the rectum if dissection is misdirected, because there may be diastasis of the vasa deferentia away from the midline.

The dissection should continue completely through the posterior bladder wall. The fatty tissue associated with the seminal vesicles and vasa deferentia will begin to appear. Once the vasa deferentia appear, they are lifted and retracted with the fourth arm. The posterior bladder neck is opened only enough to bring into view the medial edges of the seminal vesicles; opening beyond them at this time will risk injuring the neurovascular bundles prematurely. Depending on the type of procedure being performed, the technique of dissection to spare neurovascular bundles must begin at this point in the surgery.

13. SEMINAL VESICLE AND VASA DISSECTION

After the vasa and the surrounding yellow fat are dissected, the vasa are fulgurated and transected. The deferential arteries that heavily vascularize the delicate tissue associated with the vasa and seminal vesicles also must be clipped or fulgurated and transected. Once the vasa are transected, the fourth arm is used to lift one at a time to dissect and mobilize the associated seminal vesicle. Traction on the proximal end of each vas allows easier dissection to the tip of the seminal vesicles.

Having then lifted and surrounded the seminal vesicles, the surgeon must decide whether to mobilize them to their apices or transect them individually and leave the apices in situ. The latter choice is considered better for sparing nerves because it is likely to cause less trauma to the neurovascular bundle in this region.

Once mobilized or transected, the seminal vesicles and vasa must be lifted with the fourth arm. This lifting allows the surgeon access to a clean anterior layer of Denonvilliers fascia. The fourth arm is used to lift the vasa and seminal vesicles anteriorly. Movement of the rectal bougie side to side and anteriorly facilitates identification and choice of the correct area to enter for access to the cleavage plane between the rectum and prostate. Here, the surgeon must open the Denonvilliers fascia and enter the avascular plane between the rectum and prostate. The procedure also may be carried out in the plane below Denonvilliers fascia in the perirectal adipose tissue when higher volume of disease is present. To perform an oncologically sound operation and finish the case cleanly, it is crucial to complete this step slowly and carefully and to enter the correct plane.

14. NEUROVASCULAR BUNDLE DISSECTION/SPARING

In this plane, the bipolar forceps are used to spread the two structures, without the use of cautery. Placing the seminal/vasa apparatus on anterior traction clearly reveals the lateral pedicles. If it proves difficult to locate this junction, the surgeon can look laterally for the curve to find it. The rectum should be separated as much as possible from the undersurface of the prostate, especially inferolaterally toward the bundle.

Sharp dissection with scissors and a Maryland are used together to release the pedicles from the prostate. Once the pedicles are clearly apparent, the pedicle can be sectioned into small bundles, clipped, and transected. At this point, the neurovascular bundles should be released only three fourths of the distance toward the apex; the neurovascular bundle is more safely separated at the apex after the dorsal venous complex has been transected. To facilitate this dissection, the prostate can be placed on traction to the right or left.

The surgeon cleans the prostate as much as possible toward the apex from the anterior surface of the rectum by placing it on anterior traction. This placement later facilitates circumferential dissection and transection of the apical urethra. The fourth arm is now used to grasp the anterior surface of the prostate and apply slight downward and cranial traction. This traction allows the dorsal vein to be transected with minimal work, because tissue placed on traction will separate more easily. Gentle traction is the key here so as not to injure the sphincter mechanism or stretch and become misled by the length of the urethra, which will retract into the pelvis upon complete transection.

15. TRANSECTION OF THE DORSAL VENOUS COMPLEX AND URETHRA

Monopolar cautery or cold shears may be used to transect the dorsal vein until the prostatic apex and urethra are identified. A complete transection of the dorsal vein complex allows clear visualization of the prostatic apex. At this time, the surgeon works laterally to sweep the neurovascular bundles from the prostate. The fourth arm is used to roll the prostate laterally to ensure there is no apical prostatic tissue tracking posteriorly. This is the most common area for positive margins.

Once the dorsal vein is cut and the neurovascular bundles are clear, the surgeon prepares to transect the urethra sharply with the round tip scissors. A Foley catheter must be in place to recreate the circular shape of the urethra. If unable to perform more dissection posteriorly, the surgeon must be certain that the urethra can be surrounded with an instrument to ensure that it is not posteriorly tethered to the rectum. However the rectourethralis muscle may be the final tissue attachment and must be transected carefully.

16. RUNNING ANASTOMOSIS

At this point, only the anterior two thirds of the urethra is transected. The first stitch is placed outside in at the five o'clock position with a double-armed Monocryl 2-0 suture. This stitch involves tying together two 6-in. Monocryl sutures with six to seven knots by using an SH-1 or RB needle. The stitch guarantees a full thickness bite on the posterior urethra to get the anastomosis started well. Without this precaution, often it will be difficult to maintain a watertight back wall of the anastomosis and later to place the final Foley catheter.

The surgeon completes the final transection of the posterior apex with care not to cut the suture. Because this is an important area for positive margins, the surgeon must be certain to make adjustments if there was tumor at the apex on TRUS biopsy. This is also the area where Menon *(40–49)*, takes his parietal biopsies and calls a margin-based final path of this tissue regardless of the inked specimen result.

The prostate must be placed out of the surgeons vision. Normally, it is placed near the entry site of the trocar. If the specimen becomes bothersome, it may be placed in an endoretrieval bag and held out of the way. The surgeon uses the fourth arm to grab the posterior bladder neck at the four o'clock position and bring it into approximation to the urethra. The bladder neck suture is placed inside out on the bladder at the corresponding five o'clock position and at least four urethra bladder trows are made. The fourth arm is used to approximate the bladder neck and urethra, and then the sutures are cinched down in a pulley in a manner to bring the mucosal edges into contact. This procedure requires careful tension so as not to allow tearing of structures. If the bladder neck is on tension or unable to reach the urethra, the bladder may be released from the endopelvic fascia laterally and freed up anteriorly, and perineal pressure may be applied with a towel stick. It is important that the ureteric orifices not be incorporated into the anastomosis. The surgeon should always view the orifices during the anastomosis, especially when a median lobe necessitated transection of the posterior prostatovesical junction close to them. Occasionally, the bladder neck may be excessively large and may require reconstruction. Reconstruction may be performed after the posterior anastomosis is complete by placing several figure-eight sutures anteriorly to close the dog ear, or the reconstruction may need to be performed posteriorly to protect the orifices before anastomosis.

While the urethral sutures are placed, a Foley catheter is left in position to pucker out the mucosa during urethral bites. This catheter must be changed to a new Foley catheter before completing the anastomosis.

Once the left side of the anastomosis is complete and watertight, the fourth arm is used to hold gentle traction on that end of the suture to prevent loosening of the running suture. The surgeon then takes a good bite of the bladder neck outside in and then the urethra inside out at the 4 o'clock position very close to the other five o'clock suture posteriorly. Continuing the suture outside in on the bladder leads to the final anterior suture, with sutures outside of both the bladder and the urethra ready for tying. The surgeon runs up this suture and makes space on the bladder part of the anastomosis as needed.

Before the last one or two sutures are placed on the right side, the Foley catheter can be replaced with the final 18 Fr catheter and inflated to 15 cc. It is extremely important for the Foley catheter to be viewed when entering the bladder at this time before the anastomosis is completed.

The bladder is filled with 120–150 cc fluid to determine whether it is watertight. If so, the Foley catheter is removed at 6–7 days after a cystogram.

17. UNDOCKING

The surgeon bags the prostate with a small endoretrieval device and removes it via the periumbilical port site, places a #10 Jackson Pratt drain and closes the fascia of the 10- and 12-mm ports.

REFERENCES

1. Hoznek A, Menard Y, Salomon L, Abbou CC (2005) Update on laparoscopic and robotic radical prostatectomy. Curr Opin Urol 15:173–180.
2. Robinson TN, Steigmann GV (2004) Minimally invasive surgery. Endoscopy 36:48–51.
3. Phillips CK, Taneja SS, Stifelman MD (2005) Robot-assisted laparoscopic partial nephrectomy: the NYU technique. J Endourol 19:441–445, discussion 445.

4. Woo R, Lee D, Krummel TM, Albanese C (2004) Robot-assisted pediatric surgery. Am J Surg 188 (Suppl 4A):27S–37S.

5. Menon M, Hemal AK, Tewari A et al (2004) Robot-assisted radical cystectomy and urinary diversion in female patients: technique with preservation of the uterus and vagina. J Am Coll Surg 198:386–393.

6. Balaji KC, Yohannes P, McBride CL, Oleynikov D, Hemstreet GP 3rd (2004) Feasibility of robot-assisted totally intracorporeal laparoscopic ileal conduit urinary diversion: initial results of a single institutional pilot study. Urology 63:51–55.

7. Yohannes P, Puri V, Yi B, Khan AK, Sudan R (2003) Laparoscopy-assisted robotic radical cystoprostatectomy with ileal conduit urinary diversion for muscle-invasive bladder cancer: initial two cases. J Endourol 17:729–732.

8. Menon M, Hemal AK, Tewari A et al (2003) Nerve-sparing robot-assisted radical cystoprostatectomy and urinary diversion. BJU Int 92:232–236.

9. Bentas W, Wolfram M, Jones J, Brautigam R, Kramer W, Binder J (2003) Robotic technology and the translation of open radical prostatectomy to laparoscopy: the early Frankfurt experience with robotic radical prostatectomy and one-year follow-up. Eur Urol 44:175–181.

10. Wolfram M, Brautigam R, Engl T et al (2003) Robotic-assisted laparoscopic radical prostatectomy: the Frankfurt technique. World J Urol 21:128–132.

11. Cathelineau X, Rozet F, Vallancien G (2004) Robotic radical prostatectomy: the European experience. Urol Clin North Am 31:693–699.

12. Costello AJ, Haxhimolla H, Crowe H, Peters JS (2005) Installation of telerobotic surgery and initial experience with telerobotic radical prostatectomy. BJU Int 96:34–38.

13. Patel VR, Tully AS, Holmes R, Lindsay J (2005) Robotic radical prostatectomy in the community setting—the learning curve and beyond: initial 200 cases. J Urol 174:269–272.

14. Binder J, Brautigam R, Jonas D, Bentas W (2004) Robotic surgery in urology: fact or fantasy? BJU Int 94:1183–1187.

15. Ahlering TE, Skarecky D, Lee D, Clayman RV (2004) Successful transfer of open surgical skills to a laparoscopic environment using a robotic interface: initial experience with laparoscopic radical prostatectomy. J Urol 172:776–777 [comment on J Urol (2003)170:1738–1741].

16. Menon M, Shrivastava A, Tewari A et al (2002) Laparoscopic and robot-assisted radical prostatectomy: establishment of a structured program and preliminary analysis of outcomes. J Urol 168:945–949.

17. Smith JA Jr. Robotically-assisted laparoscopic prostatectomy: an assessment of its contemporary role in the surgical management of localized prostate cancer. Am J Surg 2004;188 (Suppl 4A):63S–67S.

18. Hemal AK, Menon M (2004) Robotics in urology. Curr Opin Urol 14:89–93.

19. Sandlin D (2004) Robotic-assisted prostatectomy. J Perianesth Nurs 19:114–116.

20. Gettman MT, Blute ML, Peschel R, Bartsch G (2003) Current status of robotics in urologic laparoscopy. Eur Urol 43:106–112.

21. Rassweiler J, Frede T. Robotics (2002) Telesurgery and telementoring—their position in modern urological laparoscopy. Arch Esp Urol 55:610–628.

22. Tewari A, El-Hakim A, Horninger W, Peschel R, Coll D, Bartsch G (2005) Nerve-sparing during robotic radical prostatectomy: use of computer modeling and anatomic data to establish critical steps and maneuvers. Curr Urol Rep 6:126–128.

23. Schiff JD, Mulhall JP (2005) Neuroprotective strategies in radical prostatectomy. BJU Int 95:11–14.

24. Tewari A, Peabody JO, Fischer M, Sarle R, Vallancien G, Delmas V (2003) An operative and anatomic study to help in nerve-sparing during laparoscopic and robotic radical prostatectomy. Eur Urol 43:444–454.

25. Kaouk JH, Desai MM, Abreu SC, Papay F, Gill IS (2003) Robotic-assisted laparoscopic sural nerve grafting during radical prostatectomy: initial experience. J Urol 170:909–912.

26. Gill IS, Ukimura O, Rubinstein M et al (2005) Lateral pedical control during laparoscopic radical prostatectomy: refined technique. Urology 65:23–27.

27. Ahlering TE, Eichel L, Edwards RA, Lee DI, Skarecky DW (2004) Robotic radical prostatectomy: a technique to reduce pT2 positive margins. Urology 64:1224–1228.

28. Menon M, Hemal AK, Tewari A, Shrivastava A, Bhandari A (2004) The technique of apical dissection of the prostate and urethrovesical anastomosis in robotic radical prostatectomy. BJU Int 93:715–719.

29. Lee DI, Eichel L, Skarecky DW, Ahlering TE (2004) Robotic laparoscopic radical prostatectomy with a single assistant. Urology 63:1172–1175.

30. Pick DL, Lee DI, Skarecky DW, Ahlering TE (2004) Anatomic guide for port placement for da Vinci robotic radical prostatectomy. J Endourol 18:572–575.

31. Hemal AK, Eun D, Tewari A, Menon M (2004) Nuances in the optimum placement of ports in pelvic and upper urinary tract surgery using the da Vinci robot. Urol Clin North Am 31:683–692.

32. Esposito MP, Ilbeigi P, Ahmed M, Lanteri V (2005) Use of fourth arm in da Vinci robot-assisted extraperitoneal laparoscopic prostatectomy: novel technique. Urology 66:649–652.

33. Gettman MT, Hoznek A, Salomon L et al (2003) Laparoscopic radical prostatectomy: description of the extraperitoneal approach using the da Vinci robotic system. J Urol 170:416–419.

34. Erdogru T, Teber D, Frede T et al (2004) Comparison of transperitoneal and extraperitoneal laparoscopic radical prostatectomy using match-pair analysis. Eur Urol 46:312–319.

35. Esposito M, Dakwar G, Ahmed M et al (2004) Extraperitoneal robotic prostatectomy: comparison of technique and results at one institution. J Endourol 18:691–706.

36. Joseph JV, Rosenbaum R, Madeb R, Erturk E, Patel HRH (2006) Robotic extraperitoneal radical prostatectomy: an alternative approach. J Urol 175:945–951.

37. Kattan MW, Eastham JA, Stapleton AM, Wheeler TM, Scardino PT (1998) A preoperative nomogram for disease recurrence following radical prostatectomy for prostate cancer. J Natl Cancer Inst 90:766–771.

38. Kattan MW, Wheeler TM, Scardino PT (1999) Postoperative nomogram for disease recurrence after radical prostatectomy for prostate cancer. J Clin Oncol 17:1499–1507.

39. Stephenson AJ, Scardino PT, Eastham JA et al (2005) Postoperative nomogram predicting the 10-year probability of prostate cancer recurrence after radical prostatectomy. J Clin Oncol 23:7005–7012.

40. Tewari A, Kaul S, Menon M (2005) Robotic radical prostatectomy: a minimally invasive therapy for prostate cancer. Curr Urol Rep 6:45–48.

41. Menon M, Hemal AK, the VIP Team (2004) Vattikuti Institute prostatectomy: a technique of robotic radical prostatectomy: experience in more than 1000 cases. J Endourol 18:611–619, discussion 619.

42. Menon M, Tewari A, Peabody JO et al (2004) Vattikuti Institute prostatectomy, a technique of robotic radical prostatectomy for management of localized carcinoma of the prostate: experience of over 1100 cases. Urol Clin North Am 31:701–717.

43. Menon M, Shrivastava A, Sarle R, Hemal A, Tewari A (2003) Vattikuti Institute prostatectomy: a single-term experience of 100 cases. J Endourol 17:785–790.
44. Tewari A, Menon M (2003) Vattikuti Institute prostatectomy: surgical technique and current results. Curr Urol Rep 4:119–123.
45. Menon M, Tewari A, Peabody J, VIP Team (2003) Vattikuti Institute prostatectomy: technique. J Urol 169:2289–2292.
46. Menon M, Tewari A, Vattikuti Institute Prostatectomy Team (2003) Robotic radical prostatectomy and the Vattikuti Urology Institute technique: an interim analysis of results and technical points. Urology 61(4 Suppl 1):15–20.
47. Menon M (2003) Robotic radical retropubic prostatectomy. BJU Int 91:175–176.
48. Menon M, Tewari A, Baize B, Guillonneau B, Vallancien G (2003) Prospective comparison of radical retropubic prostatectomy and robot-assisted anatomic prostatectomy: the Vattikuti Urology Institute experience. *J Urol* 170:318–319 [comment on Urology (2002)60:864–868].
49. Tewari A, Peabody J, Sarle R et al (2002) Technique of da Vinci robot-assisted anatomic radical prostatectomy. Urology 60:569–572.

SUGGESTED READINGS

Anonymous (2002) Minimally invasive procedure and robotic technology combined to treat prostate cancer. Expert Rev Anticancer Ther 2:482.

Antiphon P, Hoznek A, Benyoussef A et al (2003) Complete solo laparoscopic radical prostatectomy: initial experience. Urology 61:724–728, discussion 728–729.

Bhandari A, McIntire L, Kaul SA, Hemal AK, Peabody JO, Menon M (2005) Perioperative complications of robotic radical prostatectomy after the learning curve. J Urol 174:915–918.

Botvin JD (2004) Hartford Hospital surgeons share publicity with robot "assistants." Profiles Healthc Mark 20:1, 3–9.

Costello AJ (2005) Beyond marketing: the real value of robotic radical prostatectomy. BJU Int 96:1–2.

Eto M, Yokomizo A, Koga H et al (2005) A laparoscopic radical prostatectomy assisted by the "ZEUS" robotic system: an initial case report. Fukuoka Igaku Zasshi 96:58–62.

Hernandez DJ, Epstein JI, Trock BJ, Tsuzuki T, Carter HB, Walsh PC (2005) Radical retropubic prostatecomy. How often do experienced surgeons have positive surgical margins when there is extraprostatic extension in the region of the neurovascular bundle? J Urol 174:789–790.

Herrell SD, Smith JA Jr (2005) Laparoscopic and robotic radical prostatectomy: what are the real advantages? BJU Int 95:3–4.

Joseph JV, Vicente I, Madeb R, Erturk E, Patel HR (2005) Robot-assisted vs pure laparoscopic radical prostatecomy: are there any differences? BJU Int 96:39–42.

Lepor H, Kaci L (2003) Contemporary evaluation of operative parameters and complications related to open radical retropubic prostatectomy. Urology 62:702–706.

Lotan Y, Cadeddu JA, Gettman MT (2004) The new economics of radical prostatectomy: cost comparison of open, laparoscopic and robot-assisted techniques. J Urol 172:1431–1435.

Perer E, Lee DI, Ahlering T, Clayman RV (2003) Robotic revelation: laparoscopic radical prostatectomy by a nonlaparoscopic surgeon. J Am Coll Surg 197:693–696.

Sarle R, Tewari A, Hemal AK, Menon M (2005) Robotic-assisted anatomic radical prostatectomy: technical difficulties due to a large median lobe. Urol Int 74:92–94.

Sim HG, Yip SK, Cheng WS (2004) Re: successful transfer of open surgical skills to a laparoscopic environment using a robotic interface: initial experience with laparoscopic radical prostatectomy. J Urol 172:776–777. [comment on J Urol (2003)170:1738–1741].

Su LM, Link RE, Bhayani SB, Sullivan W, Pavlovich CP (2004) Nerve-sparing laparoscopic radical prostatectomy: replicating the open surgical technique. J Urol 173:454 [comment on Urology (2004);64:123–127.

Webster TM, Herrell SD, Chang SS et al (2005) Robotic-assisted laparoscopic radical prostatectomy versus retropubic radical prostatectomy: a prospective assessment of postoperative pain. J Urol 2005;174:912–914, discussion 914.

6 Robotic Laparoscopic Radical Cystectomy

Jay Yew and Timothy Wilson

1. INTRODUCTION

Radical cystectomy is still considered the treatment of choice for many cases of aggressive urothelial malignancy, including muscle invasion, refractory carcinoma in situ, and prostatic urethral involvement. With as many as 30-50% of T1 disease eventually progressing to muscle invasion, radical cystectomy is a reasonable treatment modality for these high-grade "superficial" cases as well *(1,2)* Furthermore, cystectomy can be considered in select nonmalignant conditions such as refractory hemorrhagic, interstitial, or radiation cystitis. For patients failing primary radiation therapy for prostate cancer *(3)* or patients with severe radiation-induced bladder neck or urethral damage, salvage cystoprostatectomy may be feasible. Minimally invasive laparoscopic techniques have already become a new gold standard for procedures such as radical nephrectomy. Currently, robotic laparoscopic approaches are being used for radical and partial nephrectomy. Benefits of robotic laparoscopic approaches to the treatment of prostate cancer are also becoming more widely accepted. The advantages of robotic laparoscopic approaches to cystectomy remain controversial. Robotic cystectomy is a considerable surgical endeavor with long operative times, significant fluid shifts, and postoperative morbidity approaching that of the open technique. However, robotic laparoscopy allows unparalleled magnified three-dimensional (3-D) vision of anatomic detail and excellent hemostasis. These features translate into significantly lower blood loss and the potential for a more efficient and meticulous anatomic radical cystectomy. As a leading center for robotic laparoscopy for urologic malignancy, the City of Hope

From: *Current Clinical Urology: Urologic Robotic Surgery*
Edited by: J. A. Stock, M. P. Esposito, and V. J. Lanteri © Humana Press, Totowa, NJ

National Medical Center has performed >3,000 robotic-assisted laparoscopic prostatectomies. Over the past 18 months, 71 robotic-assisted
laparoscopic cystectomies were performed. Overall, operative times for
robotic cystectomy averaged 6.5 h, with a mean estimated blood loss
of 600 ml. No cases required conversion to an open approach. Sixty-
three robotic cystectomies were performed for bladder cancer, with a
mean nodal count of 21. Robotic laparoscopic removal of the bladder and
prostate is technically straightforward; however, the need for a thorough
pelvic lymph node dissection makes the robotic laparoscopic radical
cystectomy highly challenging. It should probably only be undertaken by
surgeons who are already facile with the robotic laparoscopic prostatectomy and conventional open radical cystoprostatectomy.

2. SURGICAL ANATOMY CONSIDERATIONS

During robotic laparoscopic cystectomy, preserving urachal and
anterior peritoneal attachments of the bladder is useful in keeping the
bladder elevated. This facilitates access to the posterior dissection and
surgical exposure of the seminal vesicles, ureters, pelvic lymph node
regions, and bladder pedicles. In the process of dissecting the ureters
distally to their intramural entry into the bladder, the anatomy of the
vascular pedicles and lymph node dissections are nicely delineated.

Although potency results of nerve-sparing radical cystectomy are
mixed, there are described approaches that allow vascular stapling
of the posterior and lateral bladder pedicles without compromising
neurovascular bundle preservation (4). Use of the articulating laparoscopic vascular stapler, ultrasonic, and cold robotic shears, and magnified
3-D vision afford excellent opportunities to attempt neurovascular bundle
preservation.

There are understandable concerns that a minimally invasive
surgical approach may sacrifice adequacy of nodal dissection in
radical cystectomy for malignancy. A complete extended pelvic
lymphadenectomy for urothelial malignancy is crucial, and it may impart
some survival benefit, even in those patients with positive lymph node
disease. Acceptable nodal dissection should typically extend cephalad,
to above the aortic bifurcation and include presacral regions (5). This
necessitates a broader (multiquadrant) surgical field that may be difficult
to encompass with the predominant robotic technology available today.
Manual bedside adjustments of the robotic ports and arms are absolutely
necessary to allow adequate range of surgical dissection. The more
recently introduced da Vinci "S" system (Intuitive Surgical, Sunnyvale,

CA) has extended operating range and multiquadrant capabilities that may have added utility in robotic cystectomy.

Nevertheless, with expert bedside assistance and manual adjustments of the robotic arms, cystectomy can be readily performed using either current robotic systems. Using these advanced techniques, 71 robotic cystectomies have been performed at the City of Hope, with 63 patients undergoing extended nodal dissection for urothelial carcinoma of the bladder. Of these 63 cancer cases, mean nodal count was 21, which is comparable with most published open surgical series (6,7).

An orthotopic neobladder is often the preferred choice for urinary diversion. Robotic approaches are well suited for neobladder–urethral anastomosis. As demonstrated in the accompanying video, pneumoperitoneum and 3-D enhanced computer vision allow unparalleled visualization of the urethral stump and the entire anastomosis. Furthermore, proper and unobtrusive use of the fourth robotic arm down in the deep pelvis is crucial during this difficult portion of robotic cystectomy.

3. PREOPERATIVE ASSESSMENT

Before cystectomy, patients will typically have undergone transurethral resection of bladder tumor for tissue diagnosis. Bimanual examination under anesthesia also is performed before cystectomy. Further staging includes chest radiograph, computerized tomography scan of the abdomen and pelvis, and a bone scan. Routine laboratory work includes liver function tests to evaluate for any occult metastatic disease. Albumin and prealbumin levels are checked to determine any potential nutritional deficiencies. In the nutritionally depleted patient, it is usually not feasible to delay cystectomy until nutritional status improves significantly. In these cases, early postoperative institution of parenteral nutrition should be anticipated. If a colon segment urinary diversion is anticipated, a colonoscopy may be indicated to rule out any colonic disease. Patients with chronic obstructive pulmonary disease or a history of smoking will likely require pulmonary function testing. Patients of advanced age or with significant cardiac risk factors require cardiology evaluation. Morbidities of radical cystectomy can be prevented or minimized by a multidisciplinary team approach that often begins preoperatively and continues postoperatively in the intensive care unit, the surgical ward, and finally at home. If an orthotopic urinary diversion is anticipated, patients are instructed and encouraged to begin pelvic floor rehabilitation (Kegel) exercises before surgery. Within a few days before surgery, the patients are counseled by an enterostomal therapist or qualified member of the surgical team for stoma marking. Stoma marking should always be done, regardless of the anticipated urinary diversion. Patients are appropriately counseled regarding the potential need to change urinary diversion based on intraoperative findings. The day before surgery, patients complete a full mechanical and antibiotic bowel preparation either at home or as an inpatient. At our institution, we prefer to admit patients the day before surgery to ensure adequate intravenous hydration while undergoing bowel preparation. Stoma counseling and marking also is done at this time.

4. ROBOTIC INSTRUMENTATION AND OPERATING ROOM SETUP

The surgeon performing robotic radical cystectomy likely has already mastered the robotic prostatectomy. In this regard, the operating room setup and instrumentation are virtually identical to the robotic prostatectomy. Photographs of our operating room setup and port placements are included in the accompanying video. In this text, references are made to specific suture material and equipment available in our operating room. Comparable materials are readily available from a variety of manufacturers (Table 1). Some specific items mentioned include the Ethicon extra-long articulating laparoscopic stapler (ETS Flex 45) with several vascular (white) cartridge reloads for division of the lateral and posterior bladder pedicles, and at least one GI (green) cartridge for division of the dorsal vein complex. Two 8 Fr feeding tubes remain postoperatively spanning the ureteral–enteric anastomoses. At the right upper para-rectus port site, we typically place an 11/12-mm Ethicon Visiport that accommodates the extra-long laparoscopic stapler. This cephalad port position, and the articulation of the stapler, allows excellent angles for division of the lateral and posterior bladder pedicles. Robotic instrumentation is standard, with the majority of the cystectomy performed using a bipolar electrocautery Maryland dissector in the left para-rectus robotic port and a monopolar electrocautery (spatula, hook, or curved shears) in the right para-rectus robotic port. If neurovascular bundle preservation is to be performed, robotic ultrasonic shears (Olympus or Ethicon) and either the round-tip or curved robotic EndoShears are used.

5. PATIENT POSITIONING

The patient is placed in supine position on a foam or gel pad secured to the operating room table with wide cloth tape. Lower extremity sequential compression devices are placed before induction of anesthesia. After endotracheal intubation, placement of a nasogastric tube, radial arterial

Table 1
Select equipment and sutures for robotic cystoprostatectomy with planned
orthotopic (Studer) urinary diversion

Equipment and sutures	No.
Ethicon 11/12-mm port	3
Intuitive Surgical (IS) 8-mm robotic port	3
IS Bipolar Maryland dissector	1
IS Monopolar dissector (hook or spatula)	1
IS Ultrasonic shears (Olympus or Ethicon)	1
IS round-tip or curved monopolar shears	1
Stryker Flow II suction irrigator	1
Extra-long bariatric suction cannula	1
10-mm clip applier	1
5-mm EndoShears	1
Long flat graspers	2
Ethicon ETS 45 articulating extra-long stapler (45 cm)	1–2
Ethicon white vascular cartridge reloads	4-8
Ethicon green GI cartridge reloads	1–2
Ethicon laparoscopic needle drivers	2
Weck Hemo-o-Lok clip applier–large	1
Weck Hemo-o-Lok polymer clips	1 pack
16 Fr urethral (Foley) catheter	1
16 Fr red Robinson catheter	1
2-0 silk suture on SH needle	1
18–22 Fr urethral hematuria catheter	1
15 Fr round Jackson–Pratt drain (drainage end cut to 4 in.)	1
8 Fr feeding tube catheters (additional side-holes cut along catheter)	2
Ureteral drainage bags, 18-gauge blunt-tip needles, stopcocks	2
Penrose drain (0.25 in.) cut to 4 in.	2
3-0 Vicryl (violet-dyed, white undyed) on SH	2
Mini-laparotomy pads	1 pack
2-0 Vicryl on CT-3 needle	2–4
3-0 Vicryl (white undyed) on SH needle	5-8
4-0 Vicryl on RB needle	10–12
3-0 silk on SH needles (CR/pop-off)	1 pack
3-0 chromic on SH needle	1–3
Ethicon linear and TA GI staplers, with reloads	1–2
Egg-crate foam, wide cloth tape	
Stryker operating table	
Allen stirrups	
GU major open tray	
Carmalt intestinal clamp	

catheter, and central venous catheter are performed. The patient's arms are then secured at the sides with either arm boards or by tucking. The legs are placed in a low-lithotomy position with the thighs at a slight angle to the plane of the bed. The bed is then placed in steep Trendelenburg position. The egg-crate foam or gel pad prevents sliding on the table. Typically, no additional measures are required to secure the patient.

6. PORT PLACEMENTS

We use a six port configuration very similar to our robotic prosta-tectomy setup with all port sites shifted cephalad approximately 3 cm (two fingerbreadths). Shifting ports cephalad facilitates dissection of the urachus and proximal aortic, common iliac, and presacral lymph node tissues. An Ethicon 11/12-mm bladeless trocar is inserted supra-umbilically, approximately 24–26 cm from the pubic symphysis (target anatomy). This is for the robotic 3-D vision system camera arm. Three robotic operating 8-mm blunt trocars are placed at the left iliac (Pro-Grasp or Cobra), left para-rectus (bipolar Maryland), and right para-rectus (monopolar cautery) positions. The robotic para-rectus ports are placed 20–21 cm from the pubic symphysis. The left iliac robotic port is 19–20 cm from the pubic symphysis and 3 cm medial to the anterior superior iliac spine. All robotic ports and the supra-umbilical robotic camera port have at least 8–10-cm separation from each other. Two Ethicon 11/12-mm bladeless trocar assistant's ports are placed at the right iliac and upper right para-rectus (subcostal) sites. As on the left side, the right lateral iliac assistant's port is placed 19–20 cm from the pubic symphysis and 3 cm medial to the anterior superior iliac spine (see video).

7. ROBOTIC SURGICAL TECHNIQUE

7.1. Exposure and Posterior Dissection

Using sharp and electrocautery dissection, any adhesions are divided as necessary. The procedure can be initiated by incising the posterior peritoneal reflection (cul-de-sac) and entering Denonvilliers space. This exposes the posterior aspect of the bladder and prostate. However, it is often necessary and helpful to first mobilize the lateral aspect of the sigmoid colon, exposing the spermatic cord, left common iliac artery, and left ureter. This peritoneal incision should extend cephalad to at least the level of the aortic bifurcation to allow proximal dissection of the left ureter to this point. The left ureter typically requires more cephalad mobilization. Posterior dissection is started by extending the left peritoneal incision caudally and across the peritoneal reflection, anterior to the rectum.

Denonvilliers space is developed, and the rectum is dissected posteriorly, away from the seminal vesicles, vasa deferentia, and prostate. If nerve-sparing cystectomy is planned, thermal energy use is minimized with gentle blunt sweeping, ultrasonic shears or cold EndoShears dissection lateral and immediately adjacent to the seminal vesicles. Unlike in robotic radical prostatectomy, a plane anterior to the seminal vesicles is not developed. The seminal vesicles and vasa deferentia are left intact en bloc anteriorly with the prostate and bladder specimen. The rectum is swept posteriorly within Denonvilliers space in the midline as far down as possible toward the apex of prostate. It is not necessary to split and develop the plane between the layers of Denonvilliers fascia. If previously irradiated (e.g., prostate cancer salvage postradiation failure), Denonvilliers space can exhibit significant desmoplastic reaction and adherence making this dissection difficult and treacherous. If suspected based on history and digital-rectal exam, much of this posterior dissection can be done via an initial open perineal approach with subsequent closure of the perineum and continuation to robotic laparoscopy.

7.2. Left Ureter and Pelvic Lymph Node Dissection

The left ureter is identified crossing the common iliac vessels and isolated with a Penrose drain. The Penrose is clipped close to the ureter to act as a handle for gentle retraction. The ureter is mobilized down to its intramural entry into the bladder and divided between clips. A distal cross section of ureter is sent for frozen-section pathologic analysis. The left ureter is dissected proximally to allow adequate length to bring the ureter gently under the sigmoid mesentery across the presacral region to the right side. Once completely mobilized, a violet-dyed 3-0 Vicryl (color-coded) stay suture is placed and tied at the clipped end of the left ureter. Periureteral tissue is preserved as much as possible to maintain vascularity and viability of the ureter.

Using monopolar and bipolar electrocautery, nodal tissues are dissected anterior and lateral to the left common iliac artery toward the aortic bifurcation. Robotic arms and pistol-grip external setup joints may need to be shifted at this point to allow greater cephalad range of dissection (see "Special Considerations"). Nodal tissue medial to the left common iliac artery and presacral nodes may be easier to access later from the right side node dissection. The common iliac artery is followed caudally along the lateral aspect of the external iliac artery toward the femoral canal and Cloquet's node. All tissues surrounding and between the external iliac artery and vein are removed. As in open surgery, the lateral limit of dissection is the genitofemoral nerve. The distal limit is the node of Cloquet. Dissection of the bifurcation of the common iliac artery defines the lateral bladder pedicles containing the superior vesical artery and branches from the internal (hypogastric) iliac artery. The obturator nodes are accessed by first retracting the external iliac vessels medially. On the left side, this is best accomplished by the bedside assistant with the long suction/irrigator cannula or a long flat grasper. During the right-side dissection, the fourth arm Pro-Grasp is ideal for this exposure. Obturator tissues are swept medially away from the lateral pelvic sidewall until the obturator nerve and vessels are visualized. Care should be taken to look for an accessory obturator vein emptying into the external iliac vein. If present, it can usually be safely divided with bipolar electrocautery alone. Retraction of the external iliac vessels is released, and the obturator nodal dissection is then completed from the medial aspect of the external iliac vessels (as in radical prostatectomy). Obturator vessels can usually be spared, but if necessary, can be divided with bipolar electrocautery. This complete left nodal dissection, in combination with the posterior dissection, should nicely delineate the left lateral and posterior vascular pedicles of the bladder (see video).

7.3. Division of Left Bladder Pedicles

With the bladder still suspended anteriorly, orientation of the lateral pedicles may appear different from the open procedure. Lateral pedicles containing superior vesical arteries travel more posteriorly-anteriorly from the posterior-coursing internal iliac vessels. Posterior pedicles containing neurovascular bundles are medial to the lateral pedicles and can be best visualized by pushing the rectum posteriorly away from the suspended bladder. Periodically, the bladder should be emptied of urine to facilitate anterior suspension out of the field of dissection. The extra-long Ethicon articulating laparoscopic stapler via the right upper assistant's port allows excellent angles for division of pedicles bilaterally. The vascular staple cartridge reload (Ethicon ETS Flex 45 white) is used to divide the pedicles. The stapler should be articulated parallel to the rectum and positioned closer to the bladder to avoid injury to the neurovascular bundles. At this level, the neurovascular bundles should be within the posterior bladder pedicle tissues coursing alongside the rectum. Lateral and posterior pedicles may each require two to three reloads and applications of the stapler for adequate division down to the level of the endopelvic fascia. Therefore, per manufacturer recommendations, a second stapler may be required for completion of bilateral pedicles and division of the prostatic dorsal vein complex. In nerve-sparing cystectomy, ultrasonic shears and cold robotic shears also can be used at this point to further divide remaining pedicle tissue and mobilize the lateral aspect of the seminal vesicles.

7.4. Right Ureter and Pelvic Lymph Nodes

Retraction is released and the sigmoid colon is returned to the left side. The prior posterior peritoneal incision is continued to the right, lateral to the cecum and cephalad along the lateral line of Toldt. The cecum and ascending colon are mobilized and retracted medially and cephalad, exposing the spermatic cord, right ureter, and common iliac vessels. Similar to the left side, the right ureter is secured with a Penrose, mobilized down to the bladder, and divided between clips. Distal ureteral frozen section margins are taken. The right ureter typically does not require as much proximal mobilization. The distal end of the right ureter is secured using an undyed white 3-0 Vicryl (color-coded) stay suture. The bladder is emptied again to decrease size and to prevent spillage of urine later.

The robotic fourth arm from the left iliac port provides very helpful retraction during the right-side dissection. While still suspended anteriorly, the completed left-side dissection may cause the bladder to drop more and obscure the right side dissection. The fourth arm is helpful to provide additional anterior retraction of the bladder. It also nicely retracts the peritoneal incision and colon cephalad, exposing the aortic bifurcation (see video). Fourth-arm retraction frees up the assistant to provide more versatile assistance during node dissection. Right common iliac and presacral nodes are removed cephalad, up to 1–2 cm above the aortic bifurcation. Beware of the left common iliac vein crossing through the middle of this presacral region just posteromedial to left common iliac artery. Presacral tissues antero-medial to the left common iliac vessels are often easier to remove from this right-side dissection. At this time, a generous window in the sigmoid mesentery can be bluntly developed carefully to allow gentle passage of the left ureter later. The right-side nodal dissection skeletonizes the vessels from the aortic bifurcation down the common iliac vessels to the iliac bifurcation. The remainder of the external iliac and obturator dissection is identical to the left-side dissection. After the internal (hypogastric) artery, the right lateral bladder pedicles are delineated and divided with the laparoscopic vascular stapler. Additional blunt and ultrasonic dissection lateral to the seminal vesicals is done to mobilize neurovascular bundles away and expose the endopelvic fascia. At this point, the bladder specimen should be dissected entirely free posteriorly and laterally all the way down to the endopelvic fascia.

7.5. Releasing the Bladder Anteriorly

Fourth-arm retraction is released, and the bladder is dropped from the anterior abdominal fascia by incising the peritoneum just lateral to the medial umbilical ligaments using monopolar cautery. Care is taken to avoid injury to the epigastric vessels coursing laterally. This incision is carried caudal toward the open peritoneum and the exposed spermatic cord. The vas deferens is divided with monopolar cautery. The incision is continued cephalad toward the urachus. Dissection of the cephalad-most urachus requires operating very close to the camera port. This usually requires adjusting the robotic arms by pulling them out past their remote centers (see video) so that just the tips of the ports are entering the peritoneum. The camera also may need to be pulled back into the port to avoid interfering with the dissecting instruments.

The remainder of the pre-peritoneal space of Retzius is swept down bluntly to expose the anterior bladder and prostate. Endopelvic fascia is incised, as in robotic prostatectomy. Levator muscle fibers and urethral muscular sling fibers are gently swept away laterally. Bipolar and monopolar cautery are used to cauterize and sweep off excess fat off the anterior prostate and to divide the superficial dorsal vein complex.

7.6. Prostate Dissection

Puboprostatic ligaments are divided using bipolar and monopolar cautery. Additional urethral muscular sling fibers are swept away from the urethra and the dorsal vein complex fascia. Via the right upper assistant port, the Ethicon extra-long articulating laparoscopic stapler is inserted and applied to the dorsal vein complex. Using the larger GI staples (Ethicon green cartridge) allow excellent hemostasis and division of the dorsal vein complex. Before applying staples, the catheter is lubricated and moved to ensure that the urethra is not incorporated into the closed stapler. Once the catheter is moving freely, the stapler is fired and the dorsal vein complex is divided.

7.7. Prostate Neurovascular Bundle Preservation

The prostatic fascia is scored using the monopolar or bipolar electrocautery anteriorly. An appropriate neurovascular bundle-sparing interfascial plane is developed, and the fascia and neurovascular bundles are swept away laterally using blunt and sharp cold robotic EndoShears dissection. This delineated the contour of the prostate capsule. Starting at the region of the seminal vesical insertion into the base of the prostate, vascular pedicles are divided using ultrasonic shears close to the delineated prostate contour. Alternatively, pedicles can be isolated and divided between Weck polymer Hem-o-Lok clips. Remaining pedicle tissues and posterolateral neurovascular bundle attachments are swept away from the prostate using sharp dissection with robotic shears. Sharp dissection also is used to circumferentially mobilize the region of the prostate apex and urethra. Once circumferentially free, the entire specimen should be attached only by the urethra. The catheter is again checked to make sure it is in place and the bladder is empty of all urine. Optionally, the bladder may be irrigated with water and emptied at this point to minimize urine spillage into the surgical field. Using robotic shears, the anterior urethra is divided over a 16 Fr urethral catheter. The catheter is withdrawn. The posterior urethral stump is secured with a preplaced 7-in. 2-0 Vicryl suture on a CT-3 needle. This preplaced anastomotic suture is placed at the posterior 6 o'clock position and passed from inside the urethral lumen to outside. The posterior urethra is then sharply divided freeing up the entire specimen. Care is taken to avoid cutting the anastomotic Vicryl suture. The apex of the prostate is pulled up toward the camera, and the urethra is oversewn with a figure-eight 2-0 Vicryl suture on a CT-3 needle cut to 5 in. Optionally, a distal urethral margin can be excised from the specimen before oversewing and closing the urethra. The specimen is moved into the upper abdomen. The pelvis is irrigated and inspected for hemostasis. If necessary, FloSeal or Tisseel hemostatic agents are applied over the rectum and neurovascular bundles. Care is taken to secure the previously placed posterior anastomotic suture and CT-3 needle to the anterior pubic symphysis bone. A miniature laparotomy pad is inserted via the right iliac assistant port and placed down in the pelvis.

7.8. Securing the Ureters

The clipped ureters should already be secured with color-coded Vicryl stay sutures (left ureter, violet; right ureter, white). Via the right iliac assistant's port, a long flat grasper is inserted and passed under the sigmoid mesentery anterior to the aortic bifurcation. This opening was developed earlier, at the time of node dissection. The sigmoid colon is moved to the right to expose the tip of the flat grasper. The left violet stay suture is grasped and used to gently pull the tip of the left ureter under the sigmoid colon to the right side. Both ureters and stay sutures should be closely approximated at this point. The flat grasper (from the right iliac assistant port) is used to the grasp and lock on to the right white Vicryl stay suture, securing the right ureter. The grasper is kept in the right iliac port, locked-on to the right ureteral stay suture. The Pro-Grasp is removed and the robotic fourth arm is undocked and moved away from the left lateral iliac robotic port. The robotic port reducer cap is closed to prevent loss of pneumoperitoneum. A second long flat grasper is inserted. This left-side flat grasper crosses the midline to grasp and lock on to the violet-dyed left ureter stay suture. This flat grasper is also left in place in the left iliac robotic port securing the left ureter. The rest of the instruments are removed, and the robotic arms and camera are undocked from ports. The surgical cart is carefully moved back away from the patient but kept draped sterile. The specimen can be left in the upper abdomen, or now be carefully moved back down into the pelvis over the miniature laparotomy pad.

7.9. Extracorporeal Urinary Diversion

With the exception of both lateral ports, other ports are removed. Do not release or pull the flat graspers inserted in lateral iliac ports. They will be used to help locate the ureters and direct them up toward the midline incision for extracorporeal uretero-enteric anastomosis. The operating table should be kept in Trendelenburg to facilitate specimen retrieval and to prevent small intestines from falling into the pelvis. The supra-umbilical port incision is extended caudally 3–4 in. and opened up as a small midline incision. The specimen is carefully located and removed. Care is taken to avoid disrupting the anastomotic Vicryl suture or injuring the hand on the CT-3 needle down in the pelvis. The abdomen is surveyed. The liver, stomach, and retroperitoneum are palpated. Nasogastric tube position is confirmed. The lateral laparoscopic flat graspers are used to guide the ureteral stay sutures toward the hand inserted in the incision. The ureteral stay sutures are then carefully brought up into the midline incision and secured with external tonsil clamps. The flat graspers can then be released and carefully removed.

The cecum is identified and the terminal ileum is brought up into the abdominal incision. Mesenteric length and mobility is checked. Typically, if the anticipated diversion segment of ileum can be brought out of the incision and reach the pubic bone externally over the infraumbilical abdomen, without excess tension, there will be enough mobility to reach the urethral stump internally in the pelvis. Methods of urinary diversion are extensively described elsewhere in the literature (8,9). Briefly, we routinely perform a Studer orthotopic ileal neobladder. Fifteen to 20 cm of terminal ileum is preserved. Forty centimeters of ileum is marked for the neobladder. An addition 20 cm of ileum is marked for the afferent limb. In total, 60 cm of ileum is used for urinary diversion. Gastrointestinal (GI) continuity is reestablished using a standard stapled GI anastomosis. The mesenteric defect is closed to prevent internal hernias. The proximal 20 cm afferent limb is tailored with a Parker–Kerr running closure to remove the staple line. The distal 40-cm segment is detubularized and folded into a spherical configuration using a double-layer running 3-0 Vicryl closure.

7.10. Securing the Bladder Neck

The anterior closure of the neobladder should end caudally at the anticipated neobladder neck using undyed white Vicryl suture. This white Vicryl tail is left about 2 cm long as a color-coded anterior handle on the bladder neck. Posterior on the neobladder, about 3 cm above the bladder neck, a violet dyed 2-0 Vicryl suture is placed, and cut about 2–3 cm long as a posterior handle on the bladder neck. Just distal to this posterior violet Vicryl tail, a long loop of 2-0 silk suture is placed, which will later be attached to a urethral red Robinson catheter (see video).

7.11. Ureteral Reimplantation

Once the neobladder is finished, the ureters are reimplanted into the afferent limb using a 4-0 Vicryl suture interrupted anastomosis. Then, 8 Fr feeding tubes are passed up both ureters and brought out through a single puncture site in the distal afferent limb and secured with a chromic purse-string suture. By convention, the left feeding tube is cut at an oblique angle to differentiate it from the right feeding tube which is kept at a "right" angle. The feeding tubes are carefully manipulated and brought out alongside the right para-rectus robotic port and secured at the skin with a drain stitch.

The neobladder is rotated and carefully positioned along the right side. The afferent limb, ureters, and proximal pouch are pushed down into the abdomen with the bladder neck up in the lower incision. Taking care to avoid injury from the CT-3 needle, a hand is inserted into the pelvis, and the laparotomy pad is carefully removed. A 16 Fr red Robinson catheter is inserted via the urethra until it is felt in the pelvis. The tip is pulled up and out of the lower incision. The opposite end is clamped to prevent it from being pulled into the penile urethra. The tip of the catheter and the bladder neck should be in close proximity now. The 2-0 silk suture placed previously near the bladder neck is now passed thru the tip of the red catheter. This silk suture is tied as a long redundant loop and will be cut later and removed. The bladder neck is now secured to the tip of the urethral red Robinson catheter. This will be used to gently guide the bladder neck toward the urethral stump. There should now be three separate sutures available to assist in orienting, guiding, and pulling the bladder neck down to the urethra.

The entire neobladder is gently inserted back into the pelvis. Care is taken to maintain correct orientation and avoid any angulation on the afferent limb or ureters. The sigmoid colon is gently retracted to the left. The neobladder is brought down toward the urethra using a combination of hand guidance and gentle traction of the urethral red Robinson silk suture. Excess pulling or tension on the red Robinson silk suture should be avoided, because this will damage the urethra. This silk suture is used only to maintain orientation of the bladder neck and to merely guide the bladder neck toward the urethral stump.

A hand is inserted to palpate the feeding tube ureteral stents exiting the peritoneum from the right robotic port site. The robotic port is now carefully reinserted by feel alongside the exiting feeding tube ureteral stents. The hand inside the incision assists in safe passage of the robotic port without disruption of the ureteral stents. The other ports are similarly reinserted by feel at this time.

The fascia of the midline incision is closed in a running manner. A small gap is left supra-umbilically to accommodate the camera port. The Ethicon 11/12 port is inserted carefully and the abdomen is insufflated. The robotic vision system camera is inserted, and the ports and neobladder are inspected. Commonly, gas leaks from a gap around the camera port. This leak usually stops once the surgical cart is docked and the angle of the camera arm is brought down toward the horizontal plane. If persistent, surrounding the port within the incision with dry gauze or petroleum gauze can be useful. Also, the skin and subcutaneous fat can be closed around the port with wide figure-eight silk sutures or penetrating towel clamps.

7.12. Robotic Urethro-Vesical Anastomosis

Once pneumoperitoneum is re-established and the surgical cart is docked, the abdomen and pelvis are inspected. Usually, there is ample mesenteric length and the pouch will come down into the pelvis easily. If there is some tension, the fourth arm Pro-Grasp is invaluable in maintaining position of the pouch while securing the urethrovesical anastomosis. The fourth arm robotic Pro-Grasp via the left iliac port will grasp the posterior violet Vicryl suture on the bladder neck. The neobladder is then gently pulled with the fourth arm, and pushed from anterior by the bedside surgeon with a laparoscopic flat grasper to bring the bladder neck down to the urethral stump. The anterior white (undyed) Vicryl tail on the pouch suture line also is used to pull the bladder neck down. Using both the violet posterior Vicryl and the white anterior Vicryl simultaneously decreases tension on the individual sutures and avoids tearing or twisting of the neobladder. The silk suture loop connected to the urethral red Robinson should never be used to pull the pouch down, because this will cause cutting trauma to the urethra. The red Robinson catheter is slowly withdrawn as the pouch is moved down into the pelvis to guide the bladder neck toward the urethra, and to remove redundant silk suture that can get tangled with the anastomotic Vicryl suture. The robotic fourth arm is positioned alongside the lateral pelvic sidewall, and the Pro-Grasp tip is angled medially and posteriorly holding the posterior

violet suture to keep the bladder neck in place. This flush position and
the narrow profile of the robotic instruments will usually keep the fourth
arm out of the way of the other robotic instruments and camera during
anastomosis (see video). The silk suture loop between the bladder neck
and red Robinson catheter is cut and removed. The red Robinson catheter
also is removed and replaced with a 16 Fr urethral catheter. The previously placed 6-o'clock posterior suture is passed from outside to inside
at the corresponding location in the bladder neck. Meanwhile, the fourth
arm Pro-Grasp is stationary maintaining position of the bladder neck
and keeping tension off of the posterior anastomotic sutures. The 16 Fr
catheter is used to align the urethra and bladder neck and to aid in accurate
placement of urethral anastomotic sutures. It is advisable to insert at least
three posterior interrupted 2-0 Vicryl anastomotic sutures before releasing
the Pro-Grasp hold on the bladder neck. Typically, interrupted 2-0 Vicryl
sutures are placed along the posterior circumference of the anastomosis
with the suture knots on the intra-luminal side. In >3,100 robotic cases
using this anastomotic technique, there have been no episodes of stones
or bladder neck contractures attributable to intraluminal Vicryl suture
knots. The anterior anastomosis is completed with two separate running
3-0 Vicryl sutures starting at the lateral 3-o'clock and 9-o'clock positions.
These sutures are run anteriorly and tied to each other at the 12-o'clock
position. If there is any concern about tension on the anastomosis, the
entire anastomosis should be done with interrupted sutures. During the
anastomosis, the urethral catheter should be moved periodically to assure
that the catheter was not incorporated by the CT-3 needle pass. Usually,
the pouch suture line will be at this 12-o'clock position. If there is a defect
due to a larger bladder neck or from stretching, the defect can be closed
anteriorly with a separate 3-0 Vicryl suture in a figure-eight or running
closure. The pouch is irrigated via the 16 Fr urethral catheter. If there is
a leak at the anastomosis, it can usually be closed with a 3-0 Vicryl on
a smaller RB needle. Once an adequate anastomotic seal is achieved, the
16 Fr urethral catheter is removed. A new 18–22 Fr hematuria two-way
catheter is inserted easily into the neobladder. The catheter balloon is
inflated with 12-15 ml of sterile water. The neobladder is again irrigated
with the new catheter. A 15 Fr round Jackson-Pratt drain is inserted via
one of the remaining ports. The drain is positioned in the pelvis, and the
port containing the drain is carefully removed while maintaining position
of the drain. The drain is secured at the skin. The robotic surgical cart
is then undocked from the remaining ports and carefully pulled away
from the patient. The remaining ports are removed under direct vision.
The pouch orientation, ureters, drain, and feeding tube ureteral stents are
visualized before final camera removal.

8. POSTOPERATIVE MANAGEMENT

Blood loss during robotic cystectomy is typically much less than the comparable open operation. Nevertheless, operative time during robotic cystectomy can be prolonged. There can be significant fluid shifts and transient metabolic abnormalities. Intensive care, or at least monitored care, is usually warranted for the first postoperative 24 h. Central venous pressures are monitored to assist with fluid management. Nasogastric tube decompression is maintained for 24 h and then usually discontinued. Sequential pneumatic compression calf devices are mandatory at all times. The orthotopic neobladder is irrigated with normal saline every 4 h to evacuate any mucous. The feeding tube ureteral stents also are flushed with sterile saline periodically. Patients are encouraged to ambulate on postoperative day 1. Oral intake and ambulation are advanced as appropriate. If nutritionally depleted, or a prolonged ileus is anticipated, early institution of parenteral nutrition is warranted. Early in the postoperative period, the patient and family members are instructed on irrigation of the neobladder. Optionally, differential urine outputs are monitored from the urethral catheter and the individual ureteral stents. Drain outputs also are monitored and sent for creatinine measurement if urine leakage is suspected. Typically, between postoperative day 5 and day 8, increasing amounts of urine drain from the urethral catheter, and less from the ureteral stents. A stent-o-gram and pouch-o-gram (cytogram) will then be done to evaluate any potential leaks or obstruction. Stents can be removed at the bedside simultaneously or in a staged manner. The drain is typically left in place until the day after stent removal. If tolerating oral intake well and ambulating, patients can be safely discharged home before removal of ureteral stents and the drain. In patients of advanced age or with significant comorbidity or disability, early discharge planning for possible placement in appropriate rehabilitation facilities is advisable.

At home or a rehabilitation facility, the patient's neobladder should be irrigated once or twice a day to evacuate mucous. The patient typically undergoes a voiding trial and catheter removal 2 to 3 weeks after hospital discharge. Pelvic floor rehabilitation exercises are reinforced and encouraged.

9. SPECIAL CONSIDERATIONS

9.1. Specimen Removal

At the time of urinary diversion, when the supra-umbilical port incision is extended, the specimen can be removed by hand easily. Placement in a retrieval bag is not necessary. The operating table should not be moved out of Trendelenburg position because this may cause the small intestines to fall into the pelvis and obscure the specimen.

9.2. Hemostasis

Pneumoperitoneum creates an excellent working space and gently compresses tissues. This results in excellent hemostasis. Additional adjunctive techniques may include the use of Surgicel or hemostatic agents such as FloSeal and Tisseel around the areas of nodal dissection and the neurovascular bundles.

9.3. Orthotopic Neobladder Mesenteric Length

Occasionally, the mesentery of the planned diversion segment may have abundant fat or be short. This can result in a pouch that is difficult to bring down to the urethral stump. This can be anticipated at the time of extracorporeal urinary diversion by bringing the planned segment of ileum up and out of the midline incision and draping the ileum over the infra-umbilical abdominal wall. The anticipated location of the bladder neck can usually be accurately estimated. If this point on the ileum can be easily brought to the pubic symphysis or base of penis without excess tension, then typically the mesentery is generous enough to allow the orthotopic pouch to readily reach the urethral stump internally once the pouch is placed back in the pelvic. If there is still some tension when bringing the bladder down to the urethral stump, coordinated use of the three stay suture handles as well as the fourth-arm Pro-Grasp is crucial to successful anastomosis.

9.4. Urethral Anastomosis

Compared with the native bladder in a robotic prostatectomy, the ileal neobladder is typically thinner and collapsed during the anastomosis. In some cases, this may allow more room around the anastomosis. The challenge of the anastomosis is in safely bringing the bladder neck into proximity with the urethral stump without excess tension, as described above. If in doubt, it is always advisable to perform the entire anastomosis with interrupted sutures.

9.5. Fourth Arm

The fourth robotic arm (Pro-Grasp or Cobra) is crucial in robotic radical cystectomy. It is helpful in providing retraction and exposure during the pelvic lymph node dissection. It can be equally useful in maintaining position and relieving tension on the bladder neck during anastomosis. Its narrow profile and EndoWrist articulation allow it to be positioned alongside the pelvic wall unobtrusively. Without the fourth robotic arm, a second bedside assistant on the left side would be mandatory.

9.6. Port Sites and Urinary Diversion

Port sites are similar to those for prostatectomy. They are displaced a few centimeters cephalad to facilitate proximal lymph node dissection and division of the urachus. The supra-umbilical port incision is extended as a small midline incision to perform extracorporeal urinary diversion. If a noncontinent conduit is planned (e.g., Bricker or Turnbull), a conveniently located port site may be expanded and used to pull the bowel segment out to create the stoma. This should only be done if the port site coincides very closely with the preoperatively marked stoma site. A poor stoma site will cause patient dissatisfaction and easily negate any perceived benefit of using a port site for both operating and the urinary diversion. For conduits, bowel division, reanastomosis, and ureter implantation into the conduit can all be done intracorporally using robotic laparoscopic techniques. Alternatively, a small midline incision can be created for extracorporeal bowel work and conduit creation.

9.7. Collisions and Robotic Operating Reach and Range

Successful robotic surgery requires a thorough understanding of the capabilities and limitations of each robotic arm, including the camera. Furthermore, understanding the various angles of approach into the pelvis allows for proper adjustments for specific problems. These maneuvers should always be done with one hand (left hand for right-side assistant) on the port and skin entry site and the other hand (right hand) on the external handle (pistol-grip) setup joint (SUJ). Instruments should be removed from the port or pulled back near the port tip. The tips of the instrument or port must be visualized at all times during maneuvering to avoid inadvertent injury or removal of the entire port and instrument assembly out of the body.

9.8. Port Remote Center Adjustments

For problems with instrument reach and range, the entire port can be carefully pushed in or out beyond the remote center marked on each port. Pulling ports out past their remote centers allow close dissection near the camera port when dividing the urachus. Conversely, it also may be necessary to push ports in past their remote centers to allow instruments to reach the urethra down in the deep pelvis, from their more cephalad port entry sites.

9.9. External Elbow SUJ Adjustments

Moving the external handle pistol-grip setup joint caudal or cephalad can either open up or narrow the range of motion of the gray external components of each robotic arm. This translates into similar adjustments in range internally. Moving the external joint medially (toward patient) or laterally (away) also may swing the black arm assembly in or out, changing the angle of the port and instruments. To allow proximal reach above the level of the aortic bifurcation, port remote center adjustments, and external elbow SUJ angle adjustments, are usually be required. These multiple simultaneous system adjustments require a thorough understanding of the robotic instrumentation and technology and the patient's anatomy. Periodic adjustments throughout the case are usually required. Again, these maneuvers should always be done under direct vision, with one hand on the port itself at skin level, and the other hand on the external SUJ at all times, and with all instruments withdrawn into the cannula.

9.10. Arm or Pubic Bone Interference

Interference with other robotic arms or the bony pubic arch can be frustrating. It can not always be resolved completely; however, in select cases, the entire arm can be moved parallel toward the floor and medial 1–2 cm. This is done with one hand on the port at the skin entry site for stability, and the other hand at the pistol-grip SUJ near the external elbow (gray) joint. Moving the entire arm down parallel toward the floor and medial indents the abdominal skin at the port entry site, but often does not alter the remote center location intra-abdominally. This may seem like it could result in some minor added postoperative discomfort at the port site; however, this has not been observed. By moving the entire robotic arm parallel toward the floor and medial, the orientation of the instrument typically stays the same; however, the instrument's angle of approach down into the pelvis may be adjusted away from the obstructing arm or pelvic brim.

Again, while performing these maneuvers and adjustments, it is crucial to either have the instrument removed entirely, or pulled back with the dissecting tips in view at all times during maneuvering. These maneuvers are not advised or recommended by the manufacturer (Intuitive Surgical). However, with care, they can be done safely and are usually required to extend the operating range and capabilities of the surgical system during robotic cystectomy.

9.11. Female Cystectomy

Robotic cystectomy in females requires a few extra considerations. The vaginal introitus should be prepped sterile and draped to allow access intraoperatively with a vaginal retractor. This allows dissection and closure of the anterior vaginal wall if indicated. Patients also may be considered for simultaneous robotic laparoscopic colposacropexy. This technique is described elsewhere and beyond the scope of this chapter *(10)*. At our institution, women often undergo urinary diversion with a continent cutaneous stoma Indiana pouch diversion due to the higher incidence of troublesome incontinence with orthotopic neobladders in this patient population.

9.12. Obese Patients

As in open surgery, robotic cystectomy in the obese patient can be challenging. In these cases, the fourth arm and careful maneuvering of the robotic components are absolutely required. If safe, steeper Trendelenburg positioning may be helpful in allowing the intestines to fall back out of the pelvis. Extra precautions may be required in obese patients to prevent sliding. These may include additional tape across the patient and shoulder bolsters/braces attached to the head of the operating room table. Obese patients are likely to be at higher risk for postoperative thromboembolic events and wound complications. However, theoretically, wound complications in smaller laparoscopic incisions should be less likely to occur.

9.13. Prior Abdominal Surgeries

Extensive adhesions from prior operations or intra-abdominal pathology are not contraindications for robotic cystectomy. An open Hasson technique may be required for safe entry into the abdomen. In some cases, a small midline incision can be made to allow sharp dissection of bowel adherent to the anterior abdominal fascia. Once clear, the fascia can be closed to allow robotic cystectomy to proceed. The same fascial incision can be opened again later for urinary diversion. Bowel enterotomies can be closed using robotic laparoscopic techniques. Most adhesions can be divided sharply without use of thermal energy. Rarely, would adhesions require conversion to an open approach.

9.14. Urethrectomy

Urethrectomy can usually be accomplished in a similar manner to the open procedure. The patient will already be in Trendelenburg and lithotomy position. Circumferential resection of the proximal-most portion of the urethral stump can be started robotically. Once the surgical cart is undocked and pulled away, the remainder of the urethral dissection can then be completed as described previously *(8,9)*.

9.15. Respiratory Conditions

Given the recognized relationship between cigarette smoking and both bladder cancer and chronic obstructive pulmonary disease, it is not entirely uncommon to have patients with both conditions. Pneumoperitoneum can have deleterious impact on the fragile chronic obstructive pulmonary disease patient. Operating at lower insufflation pressures and adjusting minute ventilation may alleviate some of these issues.

10. MANAGEMENT OF COMPLICATIONS

Most complications of robotic radical cystectomy are identical to the comparable open approach, and management would likewise be identical. These complications include hemorrhage, rectal injury, infection, ureteroenteric stricture, parastomal hernia, incisional hernia, fistula, and bowel obstruction *(11)*.

REFERENCES

1. Esrig DE, Freeman JA, Stein JP, Skinner DG (1997) Early cystectomy for clinical stage T1 transitional cell carcinoma of the bladder. Semin Urol Oncol 15:154–160.
2. Thrasher JB, Crawford ED (1992) Minimally invasive transitional cell carcinoma (T1 and T2). In: Resnick MI, Kursh E (eds) Current therapy in genitourinary surgery, 2nd edn. BC Decker, St. Louis, Missouri, pp 74–75.
3. Bochner BH, Figueroa AJ, Skinner EC et al (1998) Salvage radical cystoprostatectomy and orthotopic urinary diversion following radiation failure. J Urol 160 :29–33.
4. Yu GW, Miller HC (eds) (1996) Critical operative maneuvers in urologic surgery. Mosby, St. Louis, Missouri.
5. Stein JP, Skinner DG (2005) The role of lymphadenectomy in high-grade invasive bladder cancer. Urol Clin North Am 2005 32:187–197.
6. Huang WC, Bochner BH (2005) Current status of establishing standards for lymphadenectomy in the treatment of bladder cancer. Curr Opin Urol 15:315–319
7. Bochner BH, Cho D, Herr HQ, Donat M, Kattan MQ, Dalbagni G (2004) Prospectively packaged lymph node dissections with radical cystectomy: evaluation of node count variability and node mapping. J Urol 172:1286–1290.
8. Hinman F Jr (ed) (1998) Atlas of urologic surgery, 2nd edn. W. B. Saunders, Philadelphia:, Pennsylvania.
9. Krane R, Siroky M, Fitzpatrick J (eds) (2000) Operative urology, 1st edn. Churchill Livingstone, New York.
10. Di Marco DS, Chow GK, Gettman MT, Elliott DS (2004) Robotic-assisted laparoscopic sacrocolpopexy for treatment of vaginal vault prolapse. Urology 63: 373–376.
11. Taneja S, Smith R, Ehrlich R (eds) (2001) Complications of urologic surgery. Prevention and management, 3rd edn. W. B. Saunders, Philadelphia, Pennsylvania.

7

Robotic Laparoscopic Nephrectomy, Partial Nephrectomy, and Nephroureterectomy

Jay Yew

1. INTRODUCTION

Solid tumors of the kidney are frequently due to renal cell carcinoma. For clinically localized renal cell carcinoma, surgical removal, via either a radical nephrectomy or a partial nephrectomy, provides the best oncologic and survival outcomes *(1–3)*. Select benign entities such as chronic pyelonephritis or marginally functioning kidneys also may be treated with surgical removal with a simple nephrectomy. The first laparoscopic nephrectomy was reported in 1991 by Clayman et al. *(4)*, and since that time, it has become the current gold standard for minimally invasive removal of the kidney. With the growing adoption of robotic technology, robotic laparoscopic surgery has expanded to include robotic nephrectomy, partial nephrectomy, and nephroureterectomy. This approach provides superior, stable, magnified three-dimensional visualization within a large transperitoneal working space. The miniature robotic instrumentation with dexterous EndoWrist range of motion provides excellent dissecting capabilities in the renal hilum. Using standardized techniques, robotic renal surgery using the da Vinci Surgical System (Intuitive Surgical, Sunnyvale, CA) can be done efficiently and safely with minimal morbidity, excellent clinical outcomes, and high patient satisfaction.

Indications for robotic radical nephrectomy include larger solid renal tumors suspicious for renal cell carcinoma. Select lesions <4 cm or exophytic lesions may be amenable to a nephron-sparing approach with

From: *Current Clinical Urology: Urologic Robotic Surgery*
Edited by: J. A. Stock, M. P. Esposito, and V. J. Lanteri © Humana Press, Totowa, NJ

a robotic partial nephrectomy. In the setting of metastatic disease, robotic nephrectomy may be indicated for intractable pain or bleeding, or for debulking before adjuvant systemic therapies. Upper tract urothelial malignancy is readily amenable to robotic laparoscopic nephroureterectomy. Contraindications to robotic laparoscopic renal surgery would include any pulmonary or cardiac conditions that would make it difficult for the patient to tolerate pneumoperitoneum. Tumor thrombus within the renal vein or vena cava also would be a contraindication.

2. PREOPERATIVE PREPARATION

The diagnosis of renal cell carcinoma is usually made with a computed tomography (CT) scan or magnetic resonance imaging. Additional staging studies may include routine laboratory studies, a chest radiograph or CT, and possibly a nuclear medicine bone scan. Multiple renal hilar vessels can sometimes be identified on standard CT imaging alone. However, more detailed three-dimensional CT angiogram reconstruction may be useful; especially before partial nephrectomy.

Patients undergoing robotic laparoscopic renal surgery should be advised of the risks of the procedure, including vascular injury, injury to adjacent organs, and the possibility of conversion to a hand-assist or open approach. The evening before surgery, patients undergo a mild bowel preparation at home with one bottle of magnesium citrate orally. Before surgery, patients are typed and crossed for 2–4 units of packed red blood cells, and receive antibiotic prophylaxis with cefazolin or a similar agent.

3. OPERATING ROOM CONFIGURATION AND PATIENT POSITIONING

The operating room is set up similarly to traditional laparoscopic renal surgery. The robotic surgical cart will typically be maneuvered toward the patient from a dorsal-cephalad direction over the ipsilateral shoulder or flank. Consequently, robotic, anesthesia, and accessory equipment (e.g., cautery generators, warmers, suction canisters) may be crowded around the head of the patient bed. Moving the patient bed to an angled orientation may facilitate organizing equipment and personnel. A clear path behind the robotic surgical cart should be maintained in the event that rapid undocking and conversion to open laparotomy is necessary. Typically, at least two monitors are available for the bedside surgeon and surgical technician. The technician's instrument table positioned near the patient's feet, with a Mayo stand over the patient's lower extremities. Before final positioning, a Foley bladder catheter and oro-gastric suction tube are placed.

The patient is placed in a full flank position, with full flexing of the table at the level of the anterior superior iliac spine. This positioning opens the angle between the costal margin and anterior superior iliac spine. The ipsilateral arm is positioned in a low praying position, close to the contralateral arm, on an airplane armrest. The table tilted in Trendelenburg position, bringing the arms toward the floor. This arm positioning and Trendelenburg table position move the ipsilateral arm maximally away and minimize interference with the cephalad external robotic arm. This positioning is especially useful in the patient with a shorter torso and narrower angle between the costal margin and anterior superior iliac spine.

4. INSTRUMENTS

Preferred instruments and materials used during robotic renal surgery are listed in Table 1 Comparable items are available from a variety of medical manufacturers. For robotic radical nephrectomy, the entire case can usually be performed with two robotic instruments: the bipolar Maryland dissector and the monopolar curved shears. The EndoWrist articulation at the tips of these robotic instruments provides the versatility and capabilities of several traditional laparoscopic instruments. These two instruments replace the monopolar hook, ultrasonic shears, bipolar paddles, shears, and a right-angle dissector. For partial nephrectomy and nephroureterectomy, two robotic needle drivers also are required during renal repair or bladder closure. If hilar vessels are to be ligated in a traditional manner using silk suture, robotic needle drivers also are required during nephrectomy.

In addition to the two standard 8-mm robotic ports, two standard 12-mm laparoscopic ports accommodate the robotic vision system camera arm and the assistant's instruments. In many cases, no additional trocars are needed. Optionally, additional 5-mm trocars can be inserted as needed. On the right side, a subxipoid midline 5-mm port allows for very effective retraction of the liver with a long locking flat grasper that reaches across and under the liver to grasp and lock-on to the lateral peritoneum and diaphragm above the liver (see video).

The assistant's 12-mm working port accommodates the laparoscopic articulating vascular stapler (ETS Flex45, Ethicon Endo-Surgery, Cincinnati, OH), 10-mm laparoscopic clip applier, and Weck Large and X-Large Hem-o-Lok clip appliers, and it allows passage of needles, sutures, and laparoscopic bulldog vascular clamps (Aesculap, Inc., Center Valley, PA). Removing this 12-mm trocar allows insertion of a large 15-mm specimen extraction bag directly through the port site

Table 1
Select equipment and sutures for robotic laparoscopic renal surgery

Item	No.	Procedure	Manufacturer
Maryland bipolar cautery dissector	1	All	Intuitive Surgical
Monopolar cautery curved endo-shears	1	All	Intuitive Surgical
Large needle drivers	2	PN, NU	Intuitive Surgical
8-mm robotic trocar/port	2	All	Intuitive Surgical
12-mm Xcel dilating trocar/port	1	All	Ethicon Endo-Surgery
12-mm bladed trocar/port	1	All	Ethicon Endo-Surgery
5-mm Xcel dilating trocar/port	1–2	All	Ethicon Endo-Surgery
5-mm locking grasper	1	All	Ethicon Endo-Surgery
5-mm endo-shears	1	All	Ethicon Endo-Surgery
5- or 10-mm ML clip applier	1	PN, NU	Ethicon Endo-Surgery
5-mm laparoscopic needle drivers	1–2	All	Ethicon Endo-Surgery
5-mm laparoscopic blunt Kitners	1–2	All	Ethicon Endo-Surgery
15-mm endo-Catch bag	1	N, NU	Ethicon Endo-Surgery
10-mm Endo-Catch Bag	1	PN	Ethicon Endo-Surgery
Laparoscopic argon beam coagulator	1	PN	
Stryker Stryke-Flow II suction/irrigator	1	All	Stryker
Carter-Thomason needlepoint passer	1	Inlet Medical	
Weck Hem-o-Lok clips (large, X-large)(and laparoscopic applier)	2–3 pk	N	Weck Closure Systems
Vessel loops (red, blue)	2	PN, NU	
1/4 in.-Penrose drain	1	PN, NU	
Lapra-Ty absorbable clips (and laparoscopic applier)	2 pk	PN	Ethicon Endo-Surgery

Laparoscopic vascular bulldog clamps (and applier and remover)	1 set	PN	Aesculap
Surgicel	1	All	Johnson & Johnson
Fibrillar	1	All	Johnson & Johnson
Avitene	1	All	Davol
FloSeal	1	PN	Baxter
Tisseel fibrin glue	1	PN	Baxter
2-0 Vicryl, CT-1 needle	4–5	PN	Ethicon Endo-Surgery
3-0 Vicryl, SH needle	2–4	PN	Ethicon Endo-Surgery
2-0 Vicryl, CT-2 or CT-3 needle	3–4	NU	Ethicon Endo-Surgery

N, nephrectomy; NU, nephroureterectomy; PN, partial nephrectomy.

incision. Additional assistant's instruments may include the following: suction/irrigator cannula, locking long flat grasper, laparoscopic endo-shears, and laparoscopic Kitners or a laparoscopic fan or paddle retractor.

For partial nephrectomy and nephroureterectomy, additional items should be available: absorbable braided sutures (2-0 and 3-0 Vicryl) and needles (SH, CT-1, and CT-2), laparoscopic needle drivers, hemostatic agents (e.g., Surgicel, Avitene, Fibrillar, FloSeal, Tisseel fibrin glue), an articulating laparoscopic ultrasound probe, and a laparoscopic argon beam coagulator.

5. TROCAR PLACEMENT

The abdomen is insufflated using an insufflation needle in the upper abdomen paramedian location. If a Hassan technique is to be used, it is usually done at the anticipated camera port location. Port sites should be planned once the abdomen is fully insufflated to 20 mmHg. Trocars are inserted with the abdomen insufflated to 20 mmHg. Robotic ports, including the robotic vision system camera port, should be spaced 8–10 cm from each other to minimize internal and external interference. The camera and cephalad robotic port sites are marked first and the placed in a longitudinal pararectus line. The cephalad trocar is marked about 2–3 cm below the costal margin, and the camera port is then measured and placed 8–10 cm below this point. Usually, this results in the camera port being lateral and cephalad to the umbilicus; however, in a shorter patient, this may require the camera port to be directly lateral to the umbilicus. Once these two ports are planned, the remaining robotic port and the assistant's working port are planned and inserted. After the camera port is inserted, the other ports are inserted under direct vision, and the insufflation is decreased to 12–15 mmHg. The caudal robotic port is placed laterally 8–10 cm from the camera port, creating a symmetrical broad V-configuration. The assistant's 12-mm working port is placed medial and caudal, usually at or below the umbilicus. This allows optimal infrahilar access to the renal hilum with either the laparoscopic stapler, clip appliers, or vascular clamps. Most cases can be done using these four ports alone. On right-sided cases, an optional midline subxiphoid 5-mm port may facilitate retraction of the liver. Optional additional ports can be placed as needed (see video).

6. NEPHRECTOMY PROCEDURE

Incising the lateral peritoneum along the line of Toldt allows medial mobilization of the colon. Peritoneal incision should be extended cephalad until either the hepatic or splenic flexures are divided. Once the peritoneum is incised, much of the colon mobilization can usually be done with gentle blunt sweeping, exposing the anterior contour of the kidney. On the right side, the duodenum is encountered, and may it initially have a similar appearance to the vena cava. The duodenum should be gently retracted medially with either a blunt Kitner, paddle or fan retractor. Duodenal attachments can be dissected sharply with cold curved shears or mobilized with gentle blunt dissection by using the cold Maryland bipolar dissector or a Kitner. Kocher mobilization of the duodenum also can be performed using the blunt-tipped monopolar spatula for gentle sweeping and minimal cautery dissection. The vena cava and right renal vein usually can be exposed posterior to the Kocherized duodenum (see video).

Once the colon is mobilized, the retroperitoneum is dissected layer-by-layer until the ureter and gonadal vessels are identified. Both can be elevated and posterior tissues dissected cephalad exposing the region of the lower pole. Once the lower pole of the kidney is mobilized and elevated, the gonadal vein can be dissected and followed cephalad to its insertion into either the vena cava (right) or renal vein (left). The gonadal vein can have considerable variation in anatomy and insertion (see video). On the right side, once the vena cava is identified, it is exposed and followed cephalad until the right renal vein is identified.

The stable, computer-enhanced three-dimensional magnified vision makes dissection of hilar structures easier and safer. The Maryland dissector is used for gentle spreading cephalad and caudal to the renal vein. Attention should be paid to the possible adrenal vein and posterior lumbar vein on the left side. On the right, the adrenal vein might be emptying into either the vena cava or the renal vein. Hilar lymphatic vessels and small accessory veins can usually be divided using the bipolar or monopolar cautery. On the left, the gonadal vein is divided between clips. If the vascular stapler is to be used, care should be taken to clip the gonadal vein well away from its insertion into the renal vein. The caudal side of the renal vein is further dissected posteriorly to identify the renal artery. Usually, the renal vein can be dissected circumferentially, which allows cephalad retraction and exposure of the renal artery posteriorly. Once the renal artery is identified and dissected, it can be clipped with either a metal clip or Weck Hem-o-Lok polymer clip (Weck Closure Systems, Research Triangle Park, NC). The artery does not need to be divided at this time. The previously dissected renal vein can now be divided using either the laparoscopic vascular stapler or multiple Hem-o-Lok polymer clips *(5)*. Before applying the stapler or clips, proper orientation and anatomic landmarks should be confirmed. For example, during right nephrectomy, check the camera horizon frequently and ensure that the vena cava is running horizontally across the bottom of the surgical field. In the left renal hilum, any arterial structures anterior to the hilum should be closely scrutinized to avoid any chance of inadvertent ligation of the superior mesenteric artery. Alternatively, using robotic techniques, a traditional ligation of the renal vein and artery by using silk suture can be performed easily. This may be a preferable technique for some surgeons due to rare reported instances of stapler malfunction *(6)* and concerns about dislodged renal artery metal clips *(7)* and recent reports of single Hem-o-Lok clip dislodgement during laparoscopic donor nephrectomies *(8)*. Once the renal vein is divided, the artery can likewise be divided, taking care to leave maximal renal artery length on the aortic side and using multiple Hem-o-Lok clips or silk suture ligatures.

Once the hilum is divided, dissection is continued directly posterior until the psoas muscle is identified. This allows easy blunt posterior dissection and elevation of Gerota's and the entire kidney specimen. In most cases, the adrenal gland can be spared. Starting at the divided hilum, a plane just caudal to the adrenal gland can usually be identified. This plane is then opened using blunt and monopolar dissection, mobilizing the upper pole of the kidney and Gerota's fascia. On the left side, this area between the hilum and the adrenal should be carefully dissected layer by layer to avoid inadvertent injury to the tail of the pancreas or splenic vessels. The previously exposed ureter is divided between clips. Finally, remaining lateral attachments to the kidney are divided, freeing up the entire specimen.

7. SPECIMEN REMOVAL

Kidney morcellation for renal cell carcinoma remains controversial. The morcellated specimen can still be evaluated for histology; however, pathologic staging is usually limited. Regardless, oncologic control and adjuvant treatment decisions are unlikely to be altered significantly by morcellation *(9)* Conversely, operative and quality of life data suggest that morcellation does not seem to significantly improve operative time, postoperative pain, or hospital stay *(10)*. Morcellation and intact removal are both acceptable practices in most cases. Removal of the umbilical 12-mm assistant's port allows insertion of a 15-mm Ethicon Endo-Catch specimen bag. Once the specimen is entrapped in the specimen bag, it can be removed by extending the umbilical port incision a few centimeters infraumbilically. Alternatively, a lower Gibson or Pfannen-stiel incision can be used for intact specimen removal. These remote site, muscle-splitting incisions may be advantageous, and they have less pain and incision-related complications *(11)*. Kidney specimen morcellation can be done manually within the specimen bag by using ring forceps. There are also several mechanical morcellators (manufactured by Karl Storz, Gynecare) that allow morcellated removal of the specimen via the umbilical port site. When morcellating the specimen, care must be taken to ensure that no adjacent organs are injured, and the specimen should be visualized throughout the morcellation procedure.

8. PARTIAL NEPHRECTOMY PROCEDURE

Regardless of tumor location, complete exposure and mobilization of the kidney are preferable to allow optimal visualization and positioning of the tumor in the middle of the surgeon's field of view. Positioning may be facilitated with mini-laparotomy pads placed under the kidney to prop up the lesion. Also, the kidney can be pulled up and positioned using temporary Vicryl suspension sutures with an absorbable Lapra-Ty clip (Ethicon Endo-Surgery) at the knot end. This suture is passed through the renal capsule at strategic locations and pulled up and passed through the abdominal wall by using the Carter-Thomason needlepoint suture-passer device (Inlet Medical, Trumbull, CT). This suture traction technique, described by Shalhav et al. *(12)* is very effective for challenging tumor locations. Once the kidney is well positioned, the lesion is imaged using intraoperative ultrasound. The capsular surface is scored with the monopolar cautery to delineate the planned excision. As in nephrectomy, the hilum is exposed completely. The hilar vessels are secured using vessel loops. Before clamping the hilar vessels, sutures are prepositioned in the surgical field or placed into the lateral or anterior abdominal wall. These sutures include premade 6-in. bolster ties of 2-0 Vicryl suture with a knot, Lapra-Ty clip, and Surgicel pledget on the end. These are used to quickly close the excision defect in the renal capsule *(12)*. Mannitol (12.5 g) is administered intravenously, and, optionally, a low-dose dopamine drip may be started. The laparoscopic bulldog vascular clamps are inserted and applied to the renal artery and vein. Using cold endo-shear dissection, the tumor is excised sharply and placed in a specimen bag. Additional deep base margins are excised separately and sent for frozen section analysis. The base of the excision is then thoroughly cauterized using the argon beam coagulator. For deeper resections of endophytic tumors, a ureteral catheter is placed preoperatively. Retrograde infusion of methylene blue is done to assess collecting system integrity. Open collecting system defects can be easily closed using 3-0 Vicryl suture on an SH needle in a figure-of-eight or running manner. Avitene (Davol Inc., Cranston, RI) or Fibrillar (Johnson & Johnson, Inc., Arlington, TX) may be preferable to Surgicel bolsters due to their powder or fluffy composition and softer compressibility. FloSeal (Baxter Inc., Deerfield, IL) also can be applied. The previously inserted 2-0 Vicryl bolster sutures are used to close the excision crater. The needle is passed widely through one edge of the capsule defect and then through the opposing edge. The suture is pulled up until the Surgicel pledget and Lapra-Ty is pulled snug against the capsule. An additional open Lapra-Ty clip and applier is inserted and used to cinch down and close the capsule snugly. The Lapra-Ty clip is then closed, securing the Vicryl bolster tie. Excessive tension is unnecessary. Once the hilar vessels are unclamped, the kidney swells, and the bolster ties become tighter. Tisseel fibrin glue (Baxter Inc.) can be liberally applied at this time to cover the area of renal repair. The hilar vessels are unclamped, and the laparoscopic bulldog vascular clamps are removed. An additional dose of mannitol (12.5 g) is administered intravenously after release of the hilar vessels. Typically, a round Jackson-Pratt closed suction drain is inserted through the lateral 8-mm robotic port site. Depending on the extent of resection and repair, an internal double-J ureteral stent may be advisable, along with Foley catheter bladder drainage to provide maximal decompression and drainage of the affected collecting system.

9. NEPHROURETERECTOMY BLADDER CUFF
PROCEDURE

Robotic-assisted laparoscopic nephroureterectomy has been previously reported *(13)*. In nephroureterectomy, various techniques have been described to address the bladder cuff in a minimally invasive manner *(14)*. Traditionally, the nephrectomy portion has been done laparoscopically (hand-assist or traditional), with the ureter and bladder cuff being addressed by a variety of techniques (open, endoscopic, laparoscopic, or combination) *(14)*. Robotic laparoscopic techniques are very well-suited for this task, and do not require any endoscopic maneuvers. Port placements are similar to those for robotic laparoscopic prostatectomy. A left iliac fourth-arm robotic port is usually not necessary. Both dissecting robotic ports are placed at the para-rectus locations, approximately 18 cm from the pubic symphysis. A right iliac 12-mm assistant's port is placed 2–3 cm medial to the anterior superior iliac spine and about 21 cm from the pubic symphysis. The robotic camera vision system 12-mm port is placed at the umbilicus. An accessory 5-mm suction/irrigator port is placed strategically in the right subcostal location. Dissection is initiated by exposing the iliac artery and following it cephalad and medial until the crossing ureter is identified. The ureter is secured with a vessel loop or Penrose drain clipped close to the ureter to allow for easy retraction on the ureter. The ureter is gently pulled cephalad and followed down to its insertion into the bladder. With gentle traction, overlying detrusor fibers are dissected exposing the intramural ureter. Once it is clear that the bladder is being tented cephalad, a generous bladder cuff is circumferentially excised. Before beginning cuff excision, the distal ureter is usually clipped to minimize spillage of urine from the involved upper tract. While retracting the ureter during cuff excision, care should be taken to avoid injuring the contralateral ureteral orifice. Indigo carmine can be administered intravenously if there is any concern about such an injury. The bladder defect is closed in multiple layers by using a running 2-0 Vicryl closure. The transected ureter is then mobilized of surrounding attachments and retracted cephalad. The Penrose or vessel loop can be left on the ureter to facilitate retrieval during the nephrectomy portion of the case. The umbilical 12-mm camera port is left in place and used as the 12-mm assistant's port during the robotic nephrectomy. During left nephroureterectomy, the 5-mm right subcostal assistant's port may be useful for insufflation or as an additional assistant's port; however, frequently it will be entrapped under bowel when the patient is repositioned in the flank position. These two ports can be left inserted in the abdomen. The other three port sites are closed in the usual manner. The two remaining ports are covered with a sterile towel stapled circumferentially around the ports. The patient is then carefully repositioned in the flank position as described above for robotic nephrectomy. Once in final flank position, the upper circumferential staples are removed, and the sterile towel is allowed to drape downward, exposing the ports. The abdomen, flank, and ports are reprepped and draped sterile in preparation for robotic laparoscopic nephrectomy. The abdomen is reinsufflated using the umbilical 12-mm port. Robotic dissecting 8-mm ports, camera 12-mm port, and any necessary assistant's 5-mm ports are placed, as described above. Nephrectomy is then performed using robotic laparoscopic techniques. Urothelial upper tract malignancy necessitates intact specimen removal within a large specimen bag. A round Jackson-Pratt drain is passed through the lateral 8-mm robotic port and positioned near the area of bladder closure.

10. POSTOPERATIVE MANAGEMENT

Nasogastric or orogastric tube decompression is usually discontinued at the conclusion of the operation. Postoperative pain control is achieved with oral or patient-controlled narcotic analgesia. In select patients, excellent pain control can be safely achieved with intravenous nonsteroidal anti-inflammatory Ketorolac as an adjunct to narcotic pain regimens (15,16). Clear liquid diet and early ambulation is initiated the evening of surgery. Urethral catheter is removed the morning after surgery. In most reasonably healthy patients, if oral intake is adequate and pain is well controlled with oral analgesics, the patient is usually discharged on the first to third postoperative day.

11. COMPLICATIONS

The stability of the three-dimensional vision system and the articulating EndoWrist instruments allows more precise dissection of the aorta, vena cava, and renal hilar vessels. This should provide greater control and minimize the incidence of vascular injury. However, in the unlikely event of injury to major veins or arteries, severe hemorrhage can result. In a hand-assist laparoscopic approach, manual compression can temporize bleeding while attempting repair or converting to open laparotomy. In robotic laparoscopic surgery, rapid conversion to open laparotomy must be planned and anticipated even before the start of the operation. This should include ensuring a clear path for rapid removal of the robotic surgical cart and having open nephrectomy surgical instruments readily available. Significant bleeding can be slowed by temporarily raising the insufflation pressure to 20–25 mmHg and gentle compression of the vascular defect with robotic instruments or a blunt Kitner or the assistant's suction/irrigator. Insertion of mini-laparotomy pads also may be useful. If venous bleeding can be controlled or slowed by robotic manipulation, the vascular injury can be repaired robotically with 3-0 silk suture or a hand-assist port can be inserted or laparotomy can be performed. If the robotic instrument is controlling bleeding, it should be left in place. Meanwhile, the operating room personnel should be preparing for laparotomy and anesthesia, providing maximal support, and calling for anticipated blood products to be immediately available. If a hand-assist port is placed, the hand can be inserted to control the bleeding while the robotic instrument is carefully moved away and removed. At this point, the robotic surgical cart can be undocked and backed away in preparation for hand-assist laparoscopic repair or open laparotomy. If bleeding can be safely slowed, then there may be an opportunity to repair vascular injuries by using previously described laparoscopic maneuvers, including the use of an occlusion balloon catheter or Foley catheter *(7,17)*. In situations where vascular injury occurs during insufflation or trocar placement, the insufflation needle or trocar should be left in place to aid in rapid localization of the site of injury. Often, conversion to open laparotomy is the most prudent course of action. In these difficult situations, promptly requesting the assistance of a vascular surgeon may be advisable and necessary.

More commonly, less severe, but significant, bleeding is encountered while dissecting the renal hilum. Frequently, this occurs when small accessory or lumbar vessels are avulsed. Often, bleeding from such vessels can be controlled or decreased with precise bipolar cautery. Small peri-hilar and peri-adrenal vessels often stop bleeding with conservative measures such as increased pneumoperitoneum, gentle compression, and hemostatic agents such as Surgicel, Avitene, or Fibrillar. Once the bleeding has ceased, the area of interest should be closely inspected and observed under low pressure (<5 mmHg) to ensure complete hemostasis. If there is ever any doubt, then it is mandatory to convert to open laparotomy to ensure adequate control of all significant vessels. The rare, but often severe, complication of major bleeding make robotic renal surgery most suitable for the experienced surgeon who is already adept at a variety of laparoscopic and robotic surgical applications.

Other complications of robotic nephrectomy parallel those of traditional laparoscopic nephrectomy and open flank nephrectomy. These complications include intraoperative bowel injuries, adjacent organ injuries (e.g., liver, spleen, and pancreas), abdominal wall or mesenteric injuries, and port site bleeding. Postoperative complications include delayed bleeding, delayed bowel perforation from thermal or unrecognized injury, intra-abdominal infection or abscess, ileus, pulmonary embolus, deep venous thrombosis, and nerve or musculoskeletal positioning injuries. The incidence and management of these complications are well described previously *(17–20)*.

12. CONCLUSIONS

Advanced robotic laparoscopic renal surgery can be performed safely, expediently, and effectively. Excellent clinical outcomes and low intraoperative morbidity require thorough understanding of relevant anatomy, operative technique, and mastery of robotic surgical maneuvers.

REFERENCES

1. Robson CJ (1963) Radical nephrectomy for renal cell carcinoma. J Urol 89:37.
2. Novick AC, Streem S, Montie JE (1989) Conservative surgery for renal cell carcinoma: a single center experience with 100 patients. J Urol 141:835.
3. Herr HW (1994) Partial nephrectomy for incidental renal cell carcinoma. Br J Urol 74:431–433.
4. Clayman RV, Kavoussi LR, Soper NJ, et al (1991) Laparoscopic nephrectomy: initial case report. J Urol 146:278–282.
5. Baumert H, Ballaro A, Arroyo C, Kaisary AV, Mulders PF, Knipscheer BC (2006) The use of polymer (Hem-o-lok) clips for management of the renal hilum during laparoscopic nephrectomy. Eur Urol 49: 816–819.
6. Chan D, Bishoff JT, Ratner L, Kavoussi LR, Jarrett TW (2000) Endovascular gastrointestinal stapler device malfunction during laparoscopic nephrectomy: early recognition and management. J Urol 164:319–321.
7. Maartense S, Heinties RJ, Idu M, Bemelman FJ, Bemelman WA (2003) Renal artery clip dislodgement during hand-assisted laparoscopic living donor nephrectomy. Surg Endosc 17:1851.
8. Meng MV (2006) Reported failures of the polymer self-locking (Hem-o-lok) clip: review of data from the Food and Drug Administration. J Endourol 20: 1054–1057.
9. Bishoff JT (2002) Laparoscopic radical nephrectomy: morcellate or leave intact? Definitely morcellate! Rev Urol 4: 34–37.
10. Varkarakis I, Rha K, Hernandez F, Kavoussi LR, Jarrett TW (2005) Laparoscopic specimen extraction: morcellation. BJU Int 95 (Suppl 2):27–31.
11. Camaroo AH, Rubenstin JN, Ershoff BD, Meng MV, Kane CJ, Stoller ML (2006) The effect of kidney morcellation on operative time, incision complications, and postoperative analgesia after laparoscopic nephrectomy. Int Braz J Urol 32: 273–279.
12. Orvieto MA, Chien GM, Tolhurst SR, et al (2005) Simplifying laparoscopic partial nephrectomy: technical considerations for reproducible outcomes. Urology 66: 976–980.
13. Nanigian DK, Smith W, Ellison LM (2006) Robot-assisted laparoscopic nephroureterectomy. J Endourol 20:463–465
14. Steinberg JR, Matin SF (2004) Laparoscopic radical nephroureterectomy: dilemma of the distal ureter. Curr Opin Urol 14:61–65
15. Freedland SJ, Blanco-Yarosh M, Sun JC et al (2002) Ketorolac-based analgesia improves outcomes for living kidney donors. Transplantation 73:741–745.

16. Diblasio CJ, Snyder ME, Kattan MW, Russo P (2004) Ketorolac: safe and effective analgesia for the management of renal cortical tumors with partial nephrectomy. J Urol 171: 1062–1065.

17. Bishoff JT, Kavoussi LR (eds) (2000) Atlas of laparoscopic retroperitoneal surgery. W.B. Saunders Company; Philadelphia, PA.

18. Bishoff JR, Allaf ME, Moore R, et al (1998) Laparoscopic bowel injuries: incidence and unique clinical presentation. J Urol 159:579.

19. Gill IBS, Kavoussi LR, Clayman RV, et al (1985) Complications of laparoscopic nephrectomy in 185 patients: a multi-institutional review. J Urol 154:479–483.

20. Taneja SS, Smith RB, Ehrlich RM (eds) (2001) Complications of urologic surgery: prevention and management, 3rd ed. W.B. Saunders Company, Philadelphia, Pennsylvania.

8   Robotic Donor Nephrectomy

María Verónica Gorodner, Carlos Galvani,
Enrico Benedetti, and Santiago Horgan

1. INTRODUCTION

Renal transplantation has emerged as the most advantageous option for the treatment of end stage renal disease. Unfortunately, despite continuing advances in medicine and technology, the increased demand for kidneys has not been followed by an increase in organ availability. The shortage of organs causes most patients to wait long periods for a transplant. In addition, there are other predictable limiting factors, such as blood type, tissue type, medical urgency, and time on the waiting list. kidney donation offers an excellent alternative to cadaveric transplantation. Based on The Organ Procurement and Transplantation Network data, >6,400 living donor transplants were performed in 2001 in the United States. In 1954, Murray performed the first successful living donor transplant between identical twins *(1)*. Since that time, hundreds of patients have received successful transplants from living donors. There are two types of living kidney donation: living related donors (e.g., sister, brother, or parents) and living nonrelated donors (e.g., wife or husband). Living donor renal transplants have demonstrated superior results compared with cadaveric grafts *(2)*.

Despite the numerous advantages offered by live donor transplants, donor nephrectomy is a major operation with no direct benefit to the donor. Moreover, when considering the technique, open nephrectomy is associated with considerable postoperative pain and lengthy recovery time *(3)*. Thus, potential donors are often hesitant to undergo this type of operation.

The increasing need for transplant organs, the associated morbidity with open donor nephrectomy, and the donor concern about postoperative

From: *Current Clinical Urology: Urologic Robotic Surgery*
Edited by: J. A. Stock, M. P. Esposito, and V. J. Lanteri © Humana Press, Totowa, NJ

pain motivated Ratner et al. to consider the laparoscopic approach as an alternative to the open technique. In 1995, Ratner performed the world's first laparoscopic live donor nephrectomy at John Hopkins Bayview Medical Center *(4)*. One year later, he reported his initial three cases. All three kidneys were transplanted successfully into the recipients, although the mean operative time was long (4 h, 6 min) *(2)*. After this initial experience, many studies reported the feasibility and safety of this technique *(5–8)*. Other studies *(9)* confirmed Ratner's hypothesis, showing that the availability of laparoscopic techniques had doubled the live donor transplantation rate, and outcomes remained excellent. Consequently, laparoscopic donor nephrectomy is currently considered standard of care. In spite of the benefits offered by laparoscopy, this technique remains associated with a steep learning curve *(10)*. Several pitfalls inherent to laparoscopic surgery can easily opaque the surgeon's performance. These pitfalls comprise an unstable video camera platform, limited motion (degrees of freedom) of straight laparoscopic instruments, two-dimensional imaging, and poor ergonomics for the surgeon *(11)*. During the past few years, an innovative technology has transformed the concept of traditional laparoscopic surgery. Robotic technology has emerged as a natural expansion of traditional laparoscopy in an attempt to reduce the technical challenges. Gill et al *(12)* were the first to report their experience performing five totally robotic nephrectomies in a porcine model. The first use of robotics in humans was at Imperial College of London in a transurethral resection of the prostate *(13)*. The da Vinci Surgical System (Intuitive Surgical, Mountain View, CA) was approved by the Food and Drug Administration in July 2000. In October 2000, we initiated our experience performing robotic hand-assisted living donor nephrectomy at our institution. In 2002, we reported our initial series with 12 patients *(14)*, and we confirmed the legitimacy of the advantages proposed for this system. The camera stability, the increased number of degrees of freedom, the three-dimensional view, and the improvement in the surgeon's ergonomics were clear advantages offered by the da Vinci Surgical System. The robotic system allows performing an accurate dissection of the renal hilum and the ureter, especially in patients with vascular abnormalities. The learning curve is relatively short, even for an inexperienced surgeon. However, robotic technology is not widely accepted due to its high costs. Another proposed downside of this system is the lack of tactile feedback. Several groups of investigators are currently working to relay touch sensation from robotic instruments back to the surgeon *(15)* Time will remedy these disadvantages.

We present our experience using the da Vinci Surgical system to perform robotic hand-assisted living related donor nephrectomy.

2. SURGICAL ANATOMY

The kidneys are retroperitoneal organs that measure approximately 11 cm in length, 6 cm in width, and 3 cm in thickness. The right kidney is positioned slightly lower than the left because of the presence of the liver. A dense fibrous capsule covers each kidney. The Gerota's fascia, a layer of connective tissue, is located between the kidneys and the psoas muscle and the lumbar spine. The perirenal fat is limited within the renal fascia, whereas the pararenal fat is located external to the fascia.

Classically, each kidney is supplied by a single renal artery and a single renal vein, arising from the abdominal aorta and entering the inferior vena cava, respectively. The left renal vein receives the left gonadal vein, the left suprarenal vein, and the left lumbar vein before crossing anterior to the aorta to join the inferior vena cava. The renal arteries typically originate off the aorta the level of L2 below the take-off of the superior mesenteric artery.

Aberrant or accessory renal arteries arise off the aorta or iliac arteries anywhere from the level of T11 to the level of L4. They are seen in up to 25% of patients. Usually, the accessory artery can be seen coursing into the renal hilum to perfuse the upper or lower polar regions. Prehilar arterial branching also is a common variant.

The most common anomaly of the left renal venous system is the circumaortic renal vein, seen in up to 15% of patients. In this anomaly, the left renal vein bifurcates into ventral and dorsal limb, which encircle the abdominal aorta. Less common is the retroaortic renal vein, seen in up to 4% of patients. Here, the single left renal vein courses posterior to the aorta and drains into the lower lumbar portion of the inferior vena cava. In addition, multiple renal veins are seen in approximately 15% of the patients.

The ureter is fibromuscular thick-walled tube, approximately 25 to 30 cm in length, with the upper half located in the abdomen and the lower half in the pelvic region. The abdominal part lies behind the peritoneum on the medial part of the psoas major, and it is crossed obliquely by the internal spermatic vessels. It enters the pelvic cavity by crossing either the termination of the common, or the commencement of the external, iliac vessels.

Proper definition of kidney vascular anatomy has traditionally been essential for planning the side of the donor nephrectomy. In the presence of normal anatomy (single artery and single vein) bilaterally, the left kidney is always preferred because of the superior length and better quality of the wall of the left renal vein.

Traditionally, the presence of multiple renal arteries was considered a contraindication to kidney transplant because of the increased risk of technical complications *(16)*. Currently, the presence of multiple arteries is not considered a contraindication to kidney procurement for transplantation, and a variety of techniques for management of multiple vessels have been described *(17)*.

The initial experience with laparoscopic procurement of the right kidney has been unfavorable because of a higher incidence of venous complications resulting in increased graft loss *(18)*. Therefore, in laparoscopic nephrectomy, it is especially important to be able to preferentially procure the left kidney.

Since the beginning of our practice, we have implemented the policy of routinely harvesting the left kidney regardless of the presence of vascular anomalies to take advantage of the longer length of the left renal vein. In our experience, the use of grafts with multiple arteries did not increase arterial or urologic complications in the recipients, and it did not affect graft survival or kidney function. We preserve the right kidney procurement for cases in which renal pathology mandates right nephrectomy for the donor's protection.

3. PREOPERATIVE ASSESSMENT

The initial assessment is performed by a transplant nurse coordinator. The patients attend an information session where they are educated about the procedure, risks and benefits. Candidates include living related donors (e.g., sister, brother, or parents) or living nonrelated donors (e.g., wife or husband). A potential donor may be considered if he or she is at least 18 years old and has a blood type compatible with the recipient. Other necessary tests include human lymphocyte antigens (HLA) tissue typing of the potential donor and a cross-match for reactive HLA. If the donor candidate is eligible, the transplant surgeon evaluates the patient. Subsequently, the potential donor is screened according to our standardized protocol (Table 1). Computed tomography (CT) angiography is the gold standard for detecting vascular anomalies, offering the opportunity of planning the surgical strategy in advance (Fig. 1).

4. INSTRUMENTATION

4.1. Robotic Instruments

- Robotic camera.
- Bipolar Maryland dissector.
- Hook electrocautery.

Table 1
Kidney donor preoperative evaluation

Transplant nurse initial assessment
- History
- Patient education session
- HLA
- ABO cross-match

Transplant surgeon
- Patient history and physical
- Review of transplant surgery

Cardiac evaluation
- Electrocardiogram
- Dobutamine stress echocardiogram >50 years

Pulmonary
- Chest X-ray.
- Pulmonary function test, if chest X-ray is abnormal

Renal
- Three urinalysis and one urine culture
- Twenty-four-h urine collection for creatinine and protein
- Double-spiral CT angiogram of abdomen three-dimensional vascular reconstruction
- Nephrology consult at surgeon's discretion

Laboratory[a]
- CBC, sickle screen (black patients), PT/PTT, Hep B Ag and Ab, hepatitis B IgG core Ab; HCV, viral serology for HSV, HZV, EBV, CMV, HIV; C3, C4, IgA, IgG, IgM, ANA, RPR; glucose, uric acid, calcium; phosphorus, liver function studies, lipid profile. Family history of diabetes requires glycosylated hemoglobin and glucose tolerance test

Psychological and social screening

Final cross-match
- One week before surgery

General surgery consultation
- With laparoscopic surgeon at least 1 week before surgery

Anesthesia evaluation

---

[a]CBC, complete blood count; PT/PTT, prothrombin time/partial thromboplastin time; Ig, immunoglobulin; Ab, antibody; HCV, hepatitis C virus; HSV, herpes simplex virus; HZV, herpes zoster virus; EBV, Epstein-Barr virus; CMV, cytomegalovirus; HIV, human immunodeficiency virus, ANA, antinuclear antibody; RPR, rapid plasma reagent.

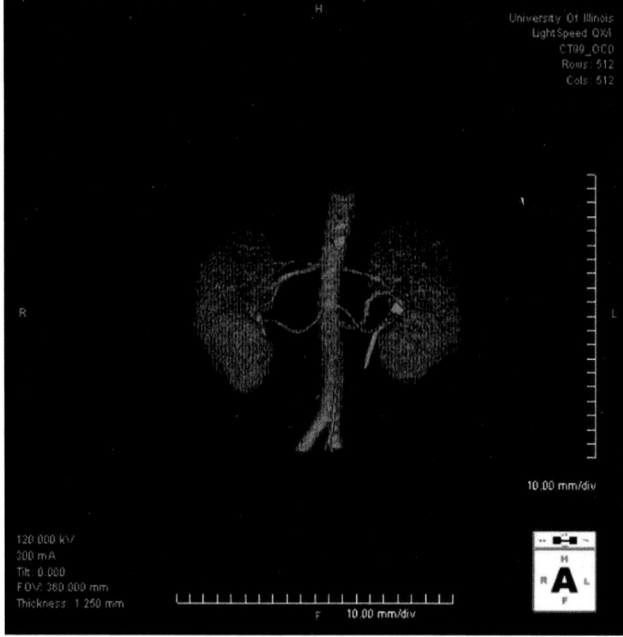

Fig. 1. CT angiography.

4.2. Laparoscopic Instruments

- Suction/irrigation.
- Grasper.
- Scissors.
- LigaSure.
- Locking clip (Hem-o-Lok Ligation System, Weck Closure Systems, Research Triangle Park, NC).
- Vascular stapler.
- Lap Disc hand port (Ethicon, Piscataway, NJ).

5. OPERATING ROOM SETUP (FIG. 2)

5.1. Robotic System (Fig. 3)

Operations are performed using the da Vinci Surgical System. This system has three components:

1. Surgeon console: The surgeon operates while seated at a console, by using four pedals, a set of console switches, and two master controls.

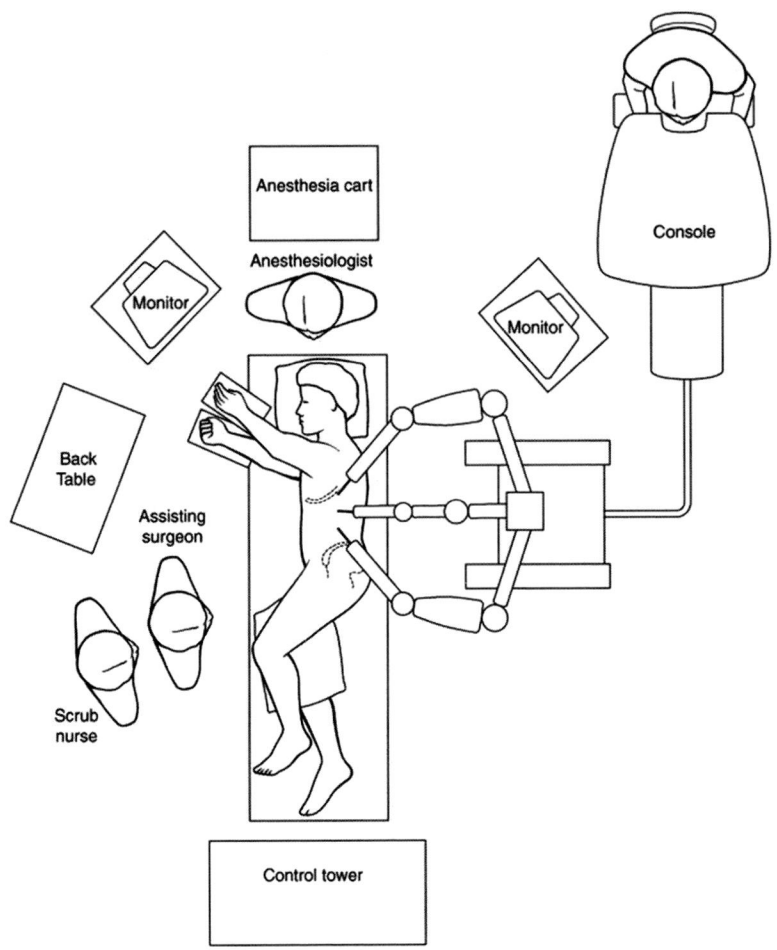

Fig. 2. Operating room setup.

The movements of the surgeon's fingers are transmitted by the master controls, to the instrument located inside the patient. A three-dimensional image of the surgical field is obtained using a 12-mm scope, which contains two cameras that integrate images.

2. Control tower: The control tower consists of a monitor, light sources, and cord attachments for the cameras.

3. Surgical arm cart: The cart provides four robotic arms, three instrument arms, and one endoscope arm, which execute the surgeon's commands.

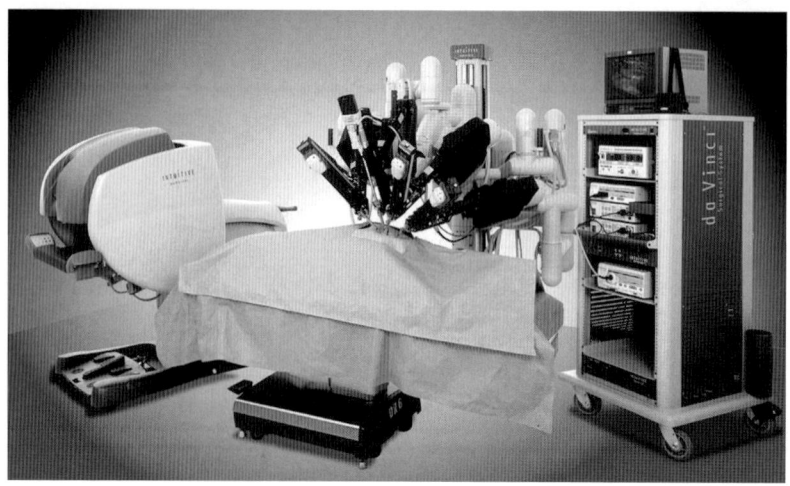

Fig. 3. Robotic system.

6. ROBOTIC HAND-ASSISTED DONOR NEPHRECTOMY

6.1. Surgical Technique

6.1.1. PATIENT POSITION

The patient is routinely positioned on a beanbag. Pneumatic compression stockings are placed on both lower extremities. Preoperative antibiotics are administered. After induction of general anesthesia, a Foley catheter and an oral gastric tube are placed. The patient is then rotated into the right lateral decubitus position with an axillary role placed under the right axilla. The beanbag is then inflated. The regular use of the beanbag permits to secure the patient to the table when the operating room table maximally flexed to open up the angle between the right costal margin and the superior iliac crest, facilitating the exposure of the kidney. Both the left arm and leg are cushioned appropriately to protect all joints and pressure points. Subsequently, the abdomen is prepped and draped in a standard sterile manner.

6.1.2. PORT PLACEMENT (FIG. 4)

A 7-cm infraumbilical midline incision is performed. A Lap Disc hand port (Ethicon) is introduced, and pneumoperitoneum is achieved with 14 mmHg CO_2 insufflation. The hand port device is used to allow the transplant surgeon to introduce his or her hand into the abdomen to facilitate retraction, dissection, and for the removal of the kidney at the end of the procedure. Under direct visualization, a 12-mm trocar is placed

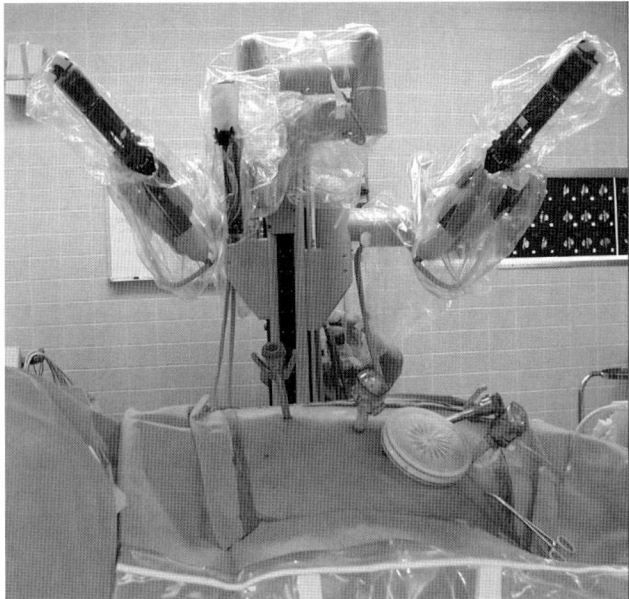

Fig. 4. Port placement.

in the supraumbilical position close to the midline. The 12-mm trocar is required for the 30° robotic camera system. Two 8-mm robotic trocars are placed, one trocar to the left of the camera trocar in the junction between the mid-clavicular line and the subcostal margin, the other trocar is placed in the mid-clavicular line to the right of the camera trocar. These two trocars are for the surgeons' right and left hand. An additional 12-mm trocar is placed in left lower quadrant, to assist with suction, clipping, stapling and cutting. The da Vinci Surgical System is then brought into position, and the arms are connected to the specific trocars.

6.1.3. Mobilization of Descending Colon and Identification of Ureter

The operation is started by mobilizing the descendent colon by incising the lateral peritoneal reflection along the first Toldt's fascia by using the hook electrocautery.

The transplant surgeons' right hand is introduced into the abdominal cavity to provide countertraction on the descending colon. The splenic flexure is taken down systematically. This maneuver allows access to the kidney. After medial rotation of the colon the psoas muscle is exposed. The ureter is identified, and it is dissected free circumferentially in a cephalad direction, beginning at the level of the left common iliac artery

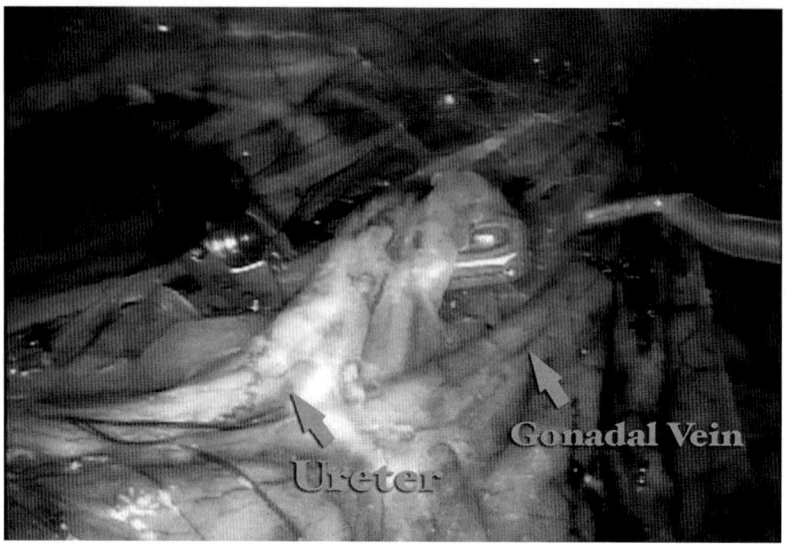

Fig. 5. Dissection of ureter.

(Fig. 5). Special attention must be taken to not harm the vasculature of the ureter. Once isolated, a 6-cm Penrose drain is introduced through the assistants' trocar to encircle the ureter. The assistant surgeon exerts lateral and anterior retraction of the ureter by grabbing the Penrose drain with a grasper.

6.1.4. POSTERIOR DISSECTION OF KIDNEY

The posterior attachments of the kidney are then taken down with the assistance of the hand of the transplant surgeon and the articulated robotic instruments. In this phase of the operation, the robot is particularly helpful in the dissection of the upper pole of the kidney from the retroperitoneal fat and the spleen, due to the articulated arm that reproduces the action of the human wrist.

6.1.5. ANTERIOR DISSECTION OF KIDNEY

The gonadal vein is identified medial to the ureter and followed superiorly up to its junction with the left renal vein. The Gerota's fascia is incised superiorly, and the kidney surface is identified. Then, following a cephalad direction, a plane between the superior medial aspect of the kidney and the adrenal gland is developed. This plane of dissection is then carried superiorly and laterally with hook cautery until the kidney is isolated from its superior pole attachments.

6.1.6. DISSECTION OF RENAL HILUM

The renal vein is circumferentially dissected using the hook cautery. Its tributaries (gonadal, lumbar, and left adrenal veins) are transected by the assistant using the LigaSure. At this point, the kidney is retracted medially, and the main renal artery and any accessory renal artery are identified and dissected free up to the level of the aortic take-off. The transplant surgeon is then able to demonstrate that the entire kidney is free from all of its attachments other than the vascular pedicles and the ureter. Once this is accomplished, the robotic system is detached from the patient, and the operation is continued laparoscopically.

6.1.7. DIVISION OF RENAL HILUM AND KIDNEY REMOVAL

The ureter is clipped twice distally at the level of the iliac artery and sharply transected by the assistant surgeon. At this point, i.v. heparin at the dose of 80 units/kg is given. Immediately after that, a locking clip (Hem-o-Lok Ligation System) is introduced by the assistant, and the renal artery is clipped at the level of the aorta take-off. The renal artery is then transected with the stapling device (vascular cartridge). The renal vein is then transected only with the stapling device. At this point, the kidney is removed through the midline incision and taken to the back table where it is flushed with cold infusion of University of Wisconsin solution (ViaSpan, Barr Laboratories, Pamona, NY). Laparoscopic inspection of the renal bed is then performed to ensure hemostasis while i.v. protamine is administered. After removal of the trocars, the midline incision is closed in one layer with a running #1 absorbable monofilament. The skin incisions are closed with subcuticular 4-0 absorbable monofilament and routinely infiltrated with 0.25% bupivacaine with epinephrine.

6.2. Special Considerations

In the presence of multiple arteries or veins, a careful back-table reconstruction is carried out by the transplant surgeon, to minimize the number of arterial or venous anastomosis to be performed in the recipient.

7. POSTOPERATIVE CARE

Patients are transferred to the floor, and they are encouraged to ambulate early. Clear liquid diet is indicated 4 to 5 h after the operation. Intravenous ketorolac and morphine are administrated for postoperative pain management. These medications are given by mouth once the patient is tolerating the diet.

A complete blood cell count, chemistry, and renal function are performed on postoperative day 1. The Foley catheter is then removed, depending on the urine output, and the results of the renal function tests. Patients are typically discharged within 2 days after the surgery.

8. MANAGEMENT OF COMPLICATIONS

8.1. Intraoperative Complications

8.1.1. VASCULAR COMPLICATIONS

The management of the vascular complications requires individual approach. At the beginning of our series, we experienced three major intraoperative bleeding. At that time, the renal artery was transected using a linear cutting vascular stapler. After experiencing three failures of the stapling device, resulting in conversion to open procedure, we modified the technique by first placing a locking clip (Hem-o-Lok, Weck Closure Systems) at the take-off of the renal artery and then dividing the artery with the stapling device. The locking clip is supposed to release the high pressure of the bloodstream, minimizing the chances of failure of the stapling device.

We believe that the use of the hand-assisted technique is critical not only to provide retraction throughout the case but also for these undesirable situations that might occur. The bleeding can be easily handled by exerting manual compression until the surgeon achieves control of the hemostasis. In case of requiring immediate conversion to open procedure, the abdominal cavity can be rapidly accessed through the already existent midline incision.

Other minor vascular injuries can occur during the dissection of the left renal vein tributaries. Lacerations or tears of the lumbar, adrenal or gonadal veins can be usually managed by applying a locking clip. If no stump is present, a 5.0 Prolene stitch should control the bleeding.

8.1.2. URETER COMPLICATIONS

Special attention must be paid to avoid damaging the vascular supply of the ureter. This is accomplished just by preserving generous amount of fat around it.

8.2. Postoperative Complications

The most frequent postoperative complications are ileus and wound infections. Less frequently, pancreatitis and pneumonia could be present. In our experience, they were all managed successfully with conservative management.

REFERENCES

1. Murray JE, Merrill JP, Harrison JH (2001) Renal homotransplantation in identical twins. 1955. J Am Soc Nephrol 12:201–204.
2. Schulam PG et al (1996) Laparoscopic live donor nephrectomy: the initial 3 cases. J Urol 155:1857–1859.
3. Simforoosh N et al (2005) Comparison of laparoscopic and open donor nephrectomy: a randomized controlled trial. BJU Int 95:851–855.
4. Ratner LE et al (1995) Laparoscopic live donor nephrectomy. Transplantation 60:1047–1049.
5. Bettschart V et al (2002) Laparoscopic procurement of kidney grafts from living donors does not impair initial renal function. Transplant Proc 34:787–790.
6. Novotny MJ (2001) Laparoscopic live donor nephrectomy. Urol Clin North Am 28:127–135.
7. Meng MV et al (2001) Laparoscopic live donor nephrectomy at the University of California San Francisco. Clin Transpl 113–121.
8. Flowers JL et al (1997) Comparison of open and laparoscopic live donor nephrectomy. Ann Surg 226:483–489, discussion 489–490.
9. Schweitzer EJ et al (1997) Increased living donor volunteer rates with a formal recipient family education program. Am J Kidney Dis 29:739–745.
10. Su LM et al (2004) Laparoscopic live donor nephrectomy: trends in donor and recipient morbidity following 381 consecutive cases. Ann Surg 240:358–363.
11. Ballantyne GH (2002) The pitfalls of laparoscopic surgery: challenges for robotics and telerobotic surgery. Surg Laparosc Endosc Percutan Tech 12:1–5.
12. Gill IS et al (2000) Robotic remote laparoscopic nephrectomy and adrenalectomy: the initial experience. J Urol 164:2082–2085.
13. Davies BL et al (1989) A surgeon robot prostatectomy—a laboratory evaluation. J Med Eng Technol 13:273–277.
14. Horgan S et al. (2002) Robotic-assisted laparoscopic donor nephrectomy for kidney transplantation. Transplantation 73:1474–1479.
15. Lanfranco AR et al (2004) Robotic surgery: a current perspective. Ann Surg 239:14–21.
16. Roza AM et al (1989) Living-related donors with bilateral multiple renal arteries. A twenty-year experience. Transplantation 47:397–399.
17. Emiroglu R et al. (2000) Multiple-artery anastomosis in kidney transplantation. Transplant Proc 32:617–619.
18. Mandal AK et al (2001) Should the indications for laparascopic live donor nephrectomy of the right kidney be the same as for the open procedure? Anomalous left renal vasculature is not a contraindiction to laparoscopic left donor nephrectomy. Transplantation 71:660–664.

9   Robotic Pyeloplasty

Jeffrey A. Stock, Michael P. Esposito,
and Gregory Lovallo

1. INTRODUCTION

The surgical treatment of ureteropelvic junction obstruction consists of two approaches. The open dismembered pyeloplasty is considered the "gold standard." More recently, minimally invasive approaches have been described, including retrograde and antegrade endopyelotomy and the Acusise procedure. These minimally invasive procedures, which involve incising the stenotic segment and placement of a stent, have not had the same success as the open procedure. The introduction of laparoscopic techniques has allowed for reproducing the steps of the open dismembered pyeloplasty while avoiding a flank incision *(1,2)*. The difficulty in mastering laparoscopic sewing has prevented the widespread use of laparoscopic pyeloplasty. The introduction of the da Vinci Surgical System (Intuitive Surgical, Sunnyvale, CA) has allowed for precision dissection and suturing. This advance has made it possible for the laparoscopic technique to reproduce the results of the open dismemberd pyeloplasty *(3)*.

2. PREOPERATIVE ASSESSMENT

Indications for laparoscopic pyeloplasty are identical to those for open pyeloplasty. Although there is considerable debate as to what constitutes absolute indications for pyeloplasty the indications for surgery should not vary based on the chosen operative technique.

Patients should undergo preoperative imaging. This imaging usually consists of ultrasonography, nuclear renal scan with diuretic washout, and voiding cystourethrogram. In some patients, the first imaging study obtained is an abdominal computed tomography (CT) scan. If a CT scan

From: *Current Clinical Urology: Urologic Robotic Surgery*
Edited by: J. A. Stock, M. P. Esposito, and V. J. Lanteri © Humana Press, Totowa, NJ

is diagnostic, we still find it useful to obtain an ultrasound and renal scan. The ultrasound provides a baseline study allowing for postoperative comparison while avoiding additional radiation exposure. The renal scan also provides differential function, which can be difficult to estimate from CT imaging.

Any patient with a history of previous abdominal surgery is at risk for abdominal adhesions. This is a relative contraindication for laparoscopic pyeloplasty. Prior surgery may alter initial port placement to prevent trocar placement through adhesions. In our experience, placement of the initial port via the open technique has allowed for safe planning of port placement and laparoscopic take-down of adhesions.

3. INSTRUMENTATION

Cystoscope 7.5 Fr, 10 Fr, 17 Fr.
Ureteral catheter 3 Fr, 4 Fr.
Double J stent 3Fr, 3.7 Fr, 4.7 Fr.
Robotic instruments: DeBakey forceps, hook cautery, round scissors, two needle drivers.
Nonrobotic instruments: suction/irrigator, 5-mm clips, Maryland dissector, 5-mm peanuts.

4. PATIENT POSITION AND PORT PLACEMENT

After retrograde stent placement, a urethral Foley catheter is inserted, and the patient is placed in a semiflank position. The patient is positioned at the edge of the table to facilitate the best angle for docking of the robotic arms.

An axillary roll is placed perpendicular to the patient. Foam or pillows are placed between the upper extremities. The patient is taped unto the table to prevent patient movement during robotic arm manipulation (Fig. 1).

Port placement is shown in Fig. 2.

5. STEP-BY-STEP APPROACH

Preoperative labs consist of complete blood count, basic metabolic profile, type and screen, and urinalysis. The patient is brought to the operating room. After general anesthesia is administered, 25 mg/kg Ancef is given. The patient is placed in the dorsal lithotomy position, and a retrograde pyelogram is obtained. We find this useful to completely define the anatomy of the ureter.

A double J stent is then placed under C-arm imaging. The length chosen should be 2 cm longer than needed. This allows for manipulation

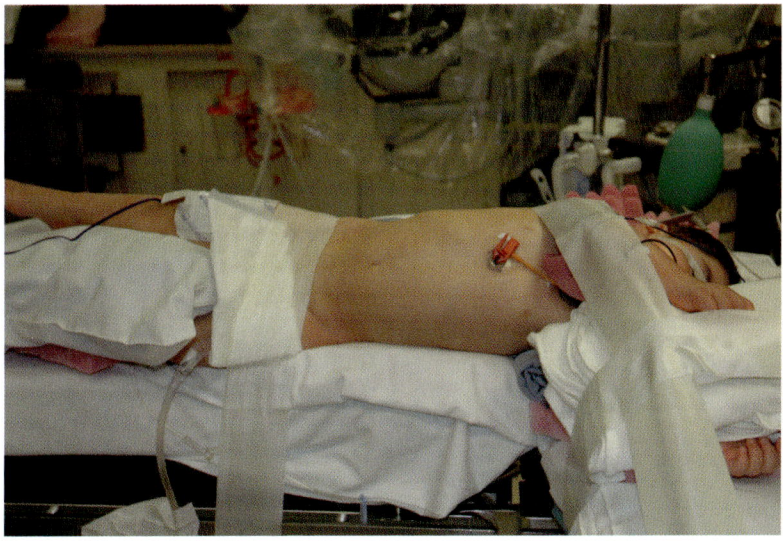

Fig. 1. Patient placement on table.

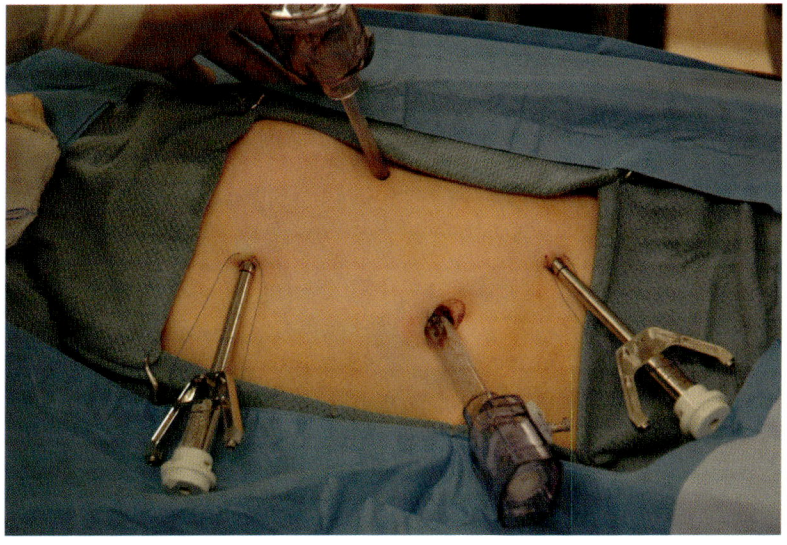

Fig. 2. Port placement.

of the proximal stent during the anastomosis while avoiding significant proximal stent migration. A Foley catheter is placed and attached to a drainage bag.

The patient is then repositioned with side of the ureteropelvic junction (UPJ) obstruction up. The kidney rest is elevated, and all pressure points are padded. A Betadine skin prep is performed. Using a Hasson technique, a 12-mm port is introduced at the superior border of the umbilicus. The 30° lens is then used to survey the abdomen. After determining that it is safe to proceed with a laparoscopic approach, three additional ports are placed. In children, we usually place two 5-mm robotic ports and one standard 5-mm port. One robotic port is placed in the midline four finger breaths above the umbilicus, and a second robotic port is placed in the lower quadrant. A third port is placed to allow for passing sutures, suction/irrigation, and retraction. It is best to place the third working port after docking the robot.

The da Vinci robot is then docked to the camera and robot arms. Dissection is started by incising the peritoneum to allow for medial retraction of the colon. This incision is accomplished using DeBakey forceps and hook cautery. It is important to identify the layers of dissection. The ureter with indwelling stent should be identified first and then traced proximally to the UPJ. Careful handling of the periureteral tissue is crucial to avoid devascularizing the ureter. If a crossing vessel is identified, then dissection must be continued proximally. The ureter is transected at the level of the UPJ, being careful not to cut the stent. The stenotic portion of ureter is excised and removed via the third working port. If crossing vessels are present, the ureter is passed anterior to the vessels and the proximal J of the stent is reintroduced into the renal pelvis.

We use 4-0 or 5-0 Vicryl suture for the anastomosis. A 9-cm length of suture is passed into the peritoneum through the third working port. Care must be taken to keep the needle in view at all times. A misplaced needle can be extremely difficult to locate.

The ureter is spatulated, and the back wall is repaired with a running suture. Next, a second stitch is used to repair the front wall. The sutures are tied together, and the needles are removed under direct laparoscopic guidance. Gerota's fascia can be loosely reapproximated with several interrupted Vicryl sutures.

The pneumoperitoneum pressure is reduced to 5 mm, and the operative area is examined to make certain that there is adequate hemostasis. The working ports are removed under laparoscopic vision. The 12-mm umbilical port is removed. All port sites are infiltrated with Marcaine. The fascia is repaired with 3-0 or 4-0 Vicryl suture. The skin is repaired with subcuticular 4-0 or 5-0 Monocryl suture.

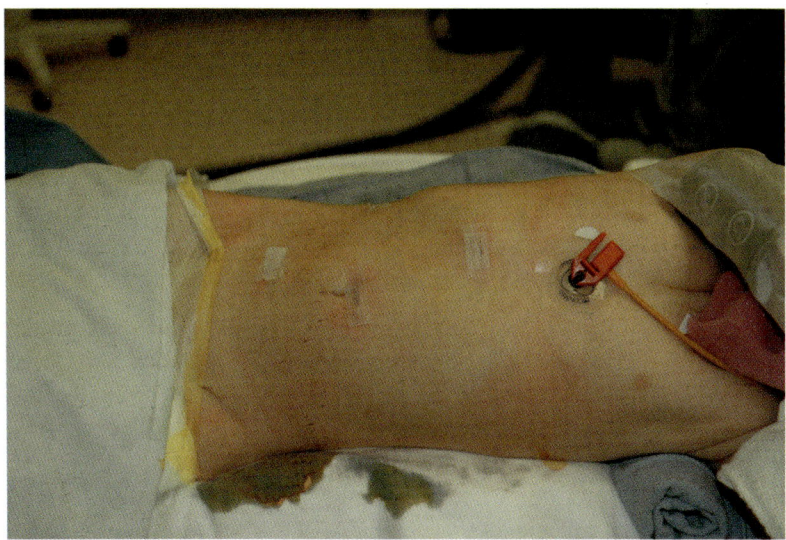

Fig. 3. Immediate post-operative appearance.

Postoperative management usually consists of intravenous Toradol (ketorolac tromethamine) for 24 h. Early in our experience, we removed the Foley catheter between 24 and 36 h postoperatively, just before hospital discharge. Most of our patients are discharged home on postoperative day 1 with an indwelling foley. The foley is removed on day 4 during the first postoperative office visit (Fig. 3).

A follow-up ultrasound is obtained 2 to 4 wk postoperatively, followed by cystoscopic removal of the stent.

6. SPECIAL CONSIDERATIONS

We prefer to place a stent cystoscopically immediately before the pyeloplasty. Other centers have reported antegrade stent placement of the stent. This can be accomplished with two different approaches.

Antegrade stent placement can be performed by placing a guide wire through one of the ports and the down the ureter. This procedure is followed by passing an appropriate diameter and length stent over the wire. An alternative approach involves percutaneous placement of a nephro-ureteo stent. This stent can be placed using a 7 Fr peel-away sheath to place a 5 Fr feeding tube through the renal pelvis, advancing the catheter through the anastomosis.

7. MANAGEMENT OF COMPLICATIONS

7.1. Intraoperative

We prefer using the Hasson technique for placement of the initial port. This technique takes additional time compared with use of the Veress needle. However difficulty with initial port placement may lead to open conversion. For difficulties related to hemostasis, please see Chap. 13.

7.2. Postoperative

Postoperative abdominal pain needs prompt evaluation. CT imaging with intravenous contrast may detect a urine leak. Delayed images taken at 3 to 4 h after injection of contrast may demonstrate a significant leak not seen on earlier delayed views. Nuclear renal scans also may demonstrate such a leak. If this leak is noted in the early postoperative period, placement of a Foley catheter to decompress the bladder and lower ureter pressure may solve the problem. If there is a large or persistent leak, then placement of a percutaneous nephrostomy tube should be considered. This approach also permits antegrade studies to evaluate the anastomosis.

Inability to complete a satisfactory anastomosis is an indication for open conversion. The possibility for open conversion should be discussed with the parents at the time informed consent is obtained.

REFERENCES

1. Kavoussi LR, Peters CA (1996) Laparoscopic pyeloplasty. J Urol 150:1891–1894.
2. Janetschek G, Peschel R, Bartasch G (1996) Laparoscopic and retroperitoneoscopic kidney pyeloplasty. Urologe A 35:202–207.
3. Atug F, Woods M, Burgess SV, Castle EP, Thomas R (2005) Robotic assisted laparoscopic pyeloplasty in children. J Urol 174:1440–1442.

10   Robotic Ureteral Reflux Surgery

Joseph G. Borer and Craig A. Peters

1. INTRODUCTION

Vesicoureteral reflux (VUR) is the retrograde flow of urine from the bladder to the upper urinary tract, and it is felt, in its primary form, to be the result of deficient submucosal tunnel length with deficient detrusor muscle backing. The prevalence of reflux in normal children has been reported to range from 1 (1) to 18.5% (2). Approximately one third of siblings of known refluxers are afflicted (3) and 67% of offspring of an affected parent (4).

In the majority of patients with reflux, the diagnosis is made during evaluation for a urinary tract infection (UTI) (5–7). However, other common reasons for evaluation for and diagnosis of vesicoureteral reflux include familial screening and prenatal hydronephrosis. Infants and younger children may present with fever, malodorous urine, dysuria, urinary frequency, lethargy, gastrointestinal symptoms, or a combination.

Any patient suspected of having reflux is placed on a prophylactic antibiotic regimen with or without an initial therapeutic antibiotic course as dictated by presentation. Antibiotic prophylaxis is continued through diagnostic evaluation that requires urethral catheterization for radio-graphic or scintigraphic study. If the diagnosis of vesicoureteral reflux is established, a management plan is formulated based on several factors, including etiology (primary vs. secondary), mode of presentation, grade of reflux, age, gender, presence of renal scarring, and general health of the patient. Early surgical intervention may be necessary for treatment of etiologic factors in patients with secondary reflux or for the treatment of primary high-grade reflux. More commonly, antibiotic prophylaxis is

From: *Current Clinical Urology: Urologic Robotic Surgery*
Edited by: J. A. Stock, M. P. Esposito, and V. J. Lanteri © Humana Press, Totowa, NJ

continued with the knowledge of expected spontaneous resolution rates, and serial examinations are performed *(5)*.

Surgical intervention for the treatment of vesicoureteral reflux should be recommended only after careful consideration of important clinical factors involved for each individual patient. Indications for early intervention include high-grade bilateral reflux or breakthrough UTI with pyelonephritis. Medical or expectant management entails a concerted effort by the patient, the patient's family, and the clinician to protect the patient from reflux-related complications such as reflux nephropathy during a period of observation until spontaneous resolution or intervention. This is the typical treatment approach for those patients with mild-to-moderate grades of reflux when spontaneous resolution is likely *(5,8,9)*. This paradigm of management may be shifting with more recent trends in endoscopic management of VUR *(10,11)*.

2. LITERATURE REVIEW

International classification system *(12)* grades I and II VUR have reported spontaneous resolution rates of 56 to 90% over 2.5 to 5 years of follow-up *(6,13–18)*. Several investigators have reported resolution of grade III reflux in approximately 50% of patients followed for up to 5 years *(16,19,20)*. In a prospective randomized investigation, patients with grades III and IV vesicoureteral reflux randomized to medical therapy were followed for 5 years in the International Reflux Study *(21)*. Reflux resolution occurred in 25% overall in 41 patients in the American arm *(22)*. In the European arm, reflux resolved in 61% with unilateral and 10% with bilateral reflux *(23)*. McLorie et al. *(20)* reported spontaneous resolution in 30% of patients with grade IV and 12% with grade V reflux followed for 5 years. VUR resolution rates have been critically reviewed and summarized *(5)*.

Numerous techniques of ureteral reimplantation have been described, but the first to receive widespread acceptance was that by Politano and Leadbetter in 1958 *(24)*. Success rates, defined as correction of vesicoureteral reflux without ureteral obstruction, have ranged from 88 to 99% for the Politano–Leadbetter ureteroneocystostomy *(25–31)*. A subsequent intravesical technique that has achieved widespread acceptance is the trans-trigonal (transverse) ureteral advancement as described by Cohen *(32)*. Excellent success rates ranging from 96 to 100% have been reported with this technique *(28,30,32–38)*.

The anatomically appealing Lich–Gregoir extravesical technique *(39,40)* was originally associated with unsatisfactory results and complication rates. A renewed interest in this less invasive approach has resulted in improved success rates ranging from 90 to 98% *(41–47)*. Modifications of the original Lich–Gregoir technique have included a combination of the ureteral orifice advancing sutures as described by Daines and Hodgson *(48)* and a more liberal circumferential detrusor dissection at the ureteral orifice described by Zaontz et al. *(49)*. Success rates incorporating these modifications have ranged from 93 to 99% *(31,49–51)*. Burbige et al. *(52)* have reported a 100% success rate in 128 children with 174 refluxing ureters using either a dismembered (64 ureters) or nondismembered (110 ureters) extravesical technique.

The first description of endoscopic treatment of VUR was by Matouschek *(53)* when he injected polytetrafluoroethylene (Teflon) paste into the subureteric region. The transurethral treatment of vesicoureteral reflux is appealing to clinicians and patients because it can be performed on an ambulatory basis, is minimally invasive, and may be highly successful. The search for the ideal injectable substance that conserves its volume and is nonmigratory and nonantigenic continues. Currently, several materials and transurethral delivery systems are in use clinically, or they are undergoing evaluation for the treatment of vesicoureteral reflux, including Teflon paste, silicone microimplants, injectable bioglass, collagen, the Deflux system, and a detachable membrane system *(54–61)*. Adequate long-term follow up assessing efficacy is still lacking for many of these injectable agents *(62)*. In addition, several autologous materials, including adipose tissue, chondrocytes, and muscle cells, have been used or are under investigation as agents for endoscopic injection to correct vesicoureteral reflux *(63)*.

The laparoscopic approach also has been applied to antireflux surgery. Techniques of dismembered *(64)*, intravesical *(65)*, and extravesical *(66–68)* approaches to laparoscopic antireflux surgery have been described previously.

Robotic ureteral reflux surgery has become an efficient and effective addition to the armamentarium of antireflux surgeries. This computer-assisted technology allows one to perform minimally invasive techniques with visual and manual acuity equal to or beyond that of open surgical techniques. This allows both surgeon and patient to avail themselves to the advantages of minimally invasive surgery with success rates comparable with those of the open technique. There is sparse literature regarding robotic-assisted laparoscopic ureteral reflux surgery. Preliminary reports include experimental *(69)* and early follow-up of clinical experience *(70)*.

3. SURGICAL ANATOMY

Pelvic anatomy is of primary interest. Care must be taken with reproductive organs and structures. The dissection in the female is chiefly between the posterior wall of the bladder and anterolateral surface of the uterus. Although dissection and extravesical reimplantation are performed in this specific area, care must be taken to avoid injury to juxtaposed structures, including the uterus, fallopian tubes, and ovaries. In boys, the vas deferens should be clearly identified along its course at the outset of the procedure, with its position continuously reviewed during the procedure.

4. PREOPERATIVE ASSESSMENT

Diagnostic evaluation is recommended after the first documented UTI with or without fever. Detection and grading of reflux are based on the appearance of radio-opaque contrast material in the upper urinary tract during voiding cystourethrogram (VCUG) according to the International Classification System established by the International Reflux Study (12). VCUG is important not only for establishing the diagnosis of reflux but also to evaluate for possible anatomic abnormality within the bladder, such as diverticula. The radionuclide cystogram (RNC) has become a staple for familial screening and follow-up of treated vesicoureteral reflux because of its increased sensitivity and decreased radiation exposure compared with VCUG, but it lacks the anatomical detail provided by VCUG. The RNC grading system correlates closely with the International Classification System (71).

Urodynamic evaluation may be indicated in children suspected of having a secondary cause for reflux (e.g., posterior urethral valves, neurogenic bladder, or non-neurogenic neurogenic bladder) as an aid both in establishing a diagnosis and guiding therapy (72–75). Cystourethroscopy has a limited role in the diagnosis of reflux, because the orthotopic ureteral orifice configuration has been found to be of little value in predicting the presence of reflux or prognosticating the likelihood of its spontaneous resolution. Cystourethroscopy is helpful before a planned extravesical approach, but it may not be necessary for those undergoing intravesical approach.

5. INSTRUMENTATION

We use the da Vinci Surgical System (Intuitive Surgical, Sunnyvale, CA). The da Vinci Surgical System includes three major components: (1) the surgeon console that contains manipulating finger controls and three-dimensional (3-D) viewing system; (2) a patient-side cart that contains the robotic working arms and 3-D endoscope; and (3) the InSite Vision System that the contains the light source, camera controls, and monitor for viewing of the operative field by operating room staff and patient-side assistant(s). Properties of this system include a master-slave robotic system, 3-D visualization of the surgical field. and fully articulating instruments.

Specific instruments used for robotic ureteral reflux surgery are listed below:

- DeBakey forceps (Intuitive Surgical)
- Electrocautery with hook (Intuitive Surgical)
- Round tip scissors (Intuitive Surgical)
- Micro forceps (Intuitive Surgical)
- 5-mm conventional laparoscopic grasping forceps
- Suction/irrigation system
- Surgical kit/instruments for open ureteral reimplantation (open and available in the operating room)

6. PATIENT POSITION

After administration of general anesthetic, the patient is placed in a dorsal lithotomy position if cystourethroscopy is to be performed. The patient is then positioned supine for robotic ureteral reflux surgery with the feet at the edge of the foot of the table. A Foley catheter is passed per urethra after the patient is prepped and draped in sterile manner. This catheter is then available for adjusting the volume of fluid (saline/urine) within the bladder to facilitate various steps of the procedure. The bladder should be evacuated of all urine at the time of trochar placement.

7. OPERATING ROOM SETUP

Operating room setup is depicted in Fig. 1. Placement of the patient, anesthesia cart, and all components of the operating room during robotic ureteral reflux surgery are depicted. This includes the da Vinci Surgical System surgeon console, the patient-side cart with 3-D endoscope, and the InSite Vision System.

8. PORT PLACEMENT

Proposed sites for port placement are shown in Fig. 2. The umbilical port is placed first via a transverse skin incision within the umbilicus. The anterior abdominal fascia is incised, and under direct vision (Hasson technique), the 12-mm cannula is passed. Alternatively, use of the Veress

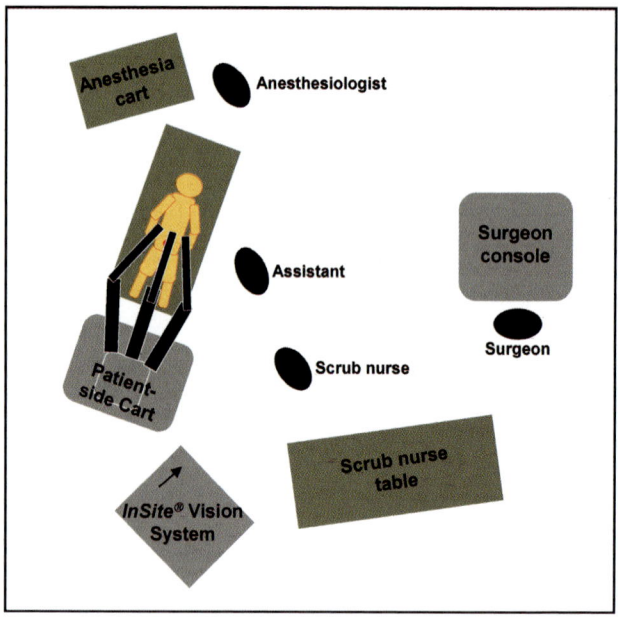

Fig. 1. Operating room set-up. Placement of the patient, anesthesia cart, and all components of the operating room during robotic ureteral reflux surgery are depicted. Not placement of the da Vinci Surgical system surgeon console, the patient-side cart with 3-D endoscope, and the InSite Vision System.

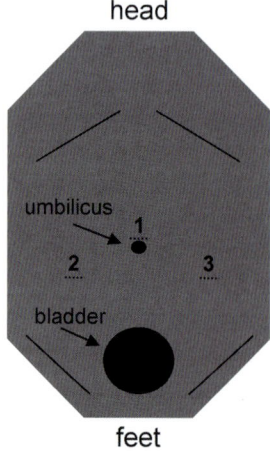

Fig. 2. Laparoscopic port placement during robotic ureteral reflux surgery are depicted. The umbilical port is placed first under direct vision (Hasson technique) the 12 mm cannula is passed or alternatively, use of the Veress needle and the Step system. The 12 mm 3-D endoscope is inserted and bilateral lower quadrant 5 mm or 8 mm instrument arm ports are placed at the mid-clavicular line under direct vision.

needle and the Step system (InnerDyne, Norwalk, CT) may be used for this initial trochar/cannula placement. The 12-mm 3-D endoscope is inserted, and the abdominal and pelvic anatomy is surveyed. Bilateral lower quadrant 5- or 8-mm instrument arm ports are placed at the mid-clavicular line on either side of midline under direct vision. The 12-mm 3-D endoscope is held and maneuvered by hand during placement of the working ports. The da Vinci Surgical system 8-mm ports are used as they specifically engage with the patient-side cart robotic instrument arms. Stay sutures of 3-O Polyglactin material may be placed in the fascia and draped over the ports to secure the ports during the procedure and approximate the fascia upon completion of the procedure.

9. STEP-BY-STEP APPROACH

After port placement and supine patient positioning, the robot is engaged. The camera port is the first to be engaged with the center arm of the patient-side cart. This is followed by passage of the camera. Working ports are then engaged to their respective trochars and instruments are safely inserted under direct vision with the 12-mm endoscope. The surgeon then assumes his or her position at the surgeon's console. Both extravesical and intravesical laparoscopic approaches have been described. The following is a step-by-step description of the extravesical technique as shown on the accompanying video.

Skin incisions are marked within the umbilicus (camera port) and over the left and right lower quadrants at the mid-clavicular line approximately three to four fingerbreadths away from and slightly (1–2 cm) caudad to the umbilicus for instrument arm trocars. After skin incision, blunt dissection with a small clamp is used to clear subcutaneous tissues down to the level of the anterior abdominal fascia. At the umbilical site, the anterior abdominal fascia is incised and under direct vision (Hasson technique) the 12-mm cannula is passed. Two simple interrupted 3-0 polyglactin sutures are then placed in the fascia to be used for securing the trochar as needed and approximation of the fascia at procedure completion. Alternatively, use of the Veress needle and the Step system may be used for this initial trochar/cannula placement. The abdominal cavity is then insufflated with CO_2 gas with pressure limit of 12–14 mmHg.

The 3-D endoscope is inserted (30° down lens) into the 12-mm trocar. Endoscopic visualization (endoscope hand-held) is used to direct insertion of the right and left lower quadrant trocars. Initial incision and blunt dissection are as per the umbilical site. A box-stitch of 3-0 polyglactin suture is then placed in the fascia to be used for securing the trochar as needed and eventual fascial closure. The trocars are passed with guidance by direct vision of the trocar point and intrabdominal contents. The robotic arms are then engaged, beginning with the camera port and followed by the two instrument ports. The camera is then inserted and attached to the robotic instrument arm. The electrocautery with hook instrument is inserted into the right robotic arm, followed by insertion of a DeBakey forceps into the left robotic arm. Under endoscopic guidance, these instruments are passed safely into position just anterior the bladder. The surgeon then moves to the surgeon's console.

At the surgeon's console, the pelvic anatomy is surveyed. Dissection begins with reflection of the peritoneum off of the bladder. The peritoneum is incised transversely beginning on the left lateral aspect of the bladder. Using primarily blunt dissection, with forceps and hook used for traction and counter traction, the distal left ureter is identified between the obliterated umbilical artery and the bladder. A stay suture is then passed through the lower abdominal wall and placed in the anterior bladder wall; 2-0 polydioxanone material is used for this traction/stay suture. This is passed under endoscopic vision through the anterior abdominal wall, passed through the bladder, and then out the anterior abdominal wall with appropriate traction applied and adjusted externally.

A detrusor trough is then created (detrusorrhaphy) on the bladder wall proximal to the ureteral insertion. Incision of detrusor fibers is carried out with either hook electrocautery or round tip scissors. A 2- to 2.5-cm detrusor incision/trough is created. Care is taken to clearly identify the bladder mucosa and avoid injury to the mucosa during this dissection. Toward completion of the detrusorrhaphy, a stay suture is passed through the anterior abdominal wall using similar material and technique as for the bladder stay suture. This is passed around the distal left ureter, and it is to be used for gentle traction on the ureter during final dissection at the ureteral insertion and during approximation of the detrusor muscle over the underlying ureter. Several simple interrupted sutures of 3-0 or 4-0 polydioxanone suture are used to approximate the detrusor muscle. These were cut in sequence with a scissors inserted through the right trocar port. A 5-mm grasping forceps was used intermittently to remove suture material and needles as appropriate.

After completion of the detrusor approximation, the caliber of the hiatus is assessed and should allow easy passage of the tips of the DeBakey forceps into the hiatus. The peritoneal lining is then approximated with a running locking suture of 4-0 polydioxanone suture. A correct needle count is ensured, and excess suture material is removed. The robot patient-side cart is disengaged from the trochars and moved away from the patient. Instrument arm ports are removed under direct vision with the hand-held endoscope followed by removal of the endoscope itself. Incisions are closed beginning with the tying of the 3-0 polyglactin sutures previously placed in the anterior abdominal wall fascia, followed by approximation of subcutaneous tissue and skin. Skin incisions are dressed with adhesive strips, absorbent dressing, and transparent adhesive cover. The patient is managed with oral analgesics and discharged home after a 1–2-day observation period.

10. SPECIAL CONSIDERATION (HEMOSTASIS)

Hemostasis is achieved when necessary with fine application of electrocautery by using the electrocautery with hook instrument. At completion of the procedure, the integrity of the bladder mucosa is checked by saline fill of the bladder via the indwelling Foley urethral catheter. At this time, surgical sites on the bladder should be directly observed for any evidence of extravasation.

11. MANAGEMENT OF COMPLICATIONS

Potential intraoperative complications include urinary extravasation/bladder injury, excessive bleeding, ureteral injury, and pelvic organ injury. Urinary extravasation after extravesical reflux surgery should be treated with indwelling Foley catheter per urethra. This management is also used for urinary retention that may occur in bilateral extravesical ureteral reimplantation.

REFERENCES

1. Arant BS Jr (1991) Vesicoureteric reflux and renal injury. Am J Kidney Dis 17:491–511.
2. Köllerman VMW (1974) Uberbewertung der pathogenetischen bedeutung des visiko-ureteralen refluxes im kindesalter. Zschr Urol 67:573–577.
3. Connolly LP, Treves ST, Zurakowski D, Bauer SB (1996) Natural history of vesicoureteral reflux in siblings. J Urol 156:1805–1807.
4. Noe HN, Wyatt RJ, Peeden JN Jr, Rivas ML (1992) The transmission of vesicoureteral reflux from parent to child. J Urol 148:1869–1871.
5. Elder JS, Peters CA, Arant BS Jr et al (1997) Pediatric Vesicoureteral Reflux Guidelines Panel summary report on the management of primary vesicoureteral reflux in children. J Urol 157:1846–1851.
6. Greenfield SP, Ng M, Wan J (1997) Experience with vesicoureteral reflux in children: clinical characteristics. J Urol 158:574–577.
7. Practice parameter: the diagnosis, treatment, and evaluation of the initial urinary tract infection in febrile infants and young children. American Academy of Pediatrics. Committee on Quality Improvement. Subcommittee on Urinary Tract Infection [published errata appear in Pediatrics 1999 May;103(5 Pt 1):1052, 1999 Jul;104(1 Pt 1):118 and 2000 Jan;105(1 Pt 1):141] [see comments]. Pediatrics 1999; 103(4 Pt 1):843–52.

8. Elder JS (2005) Imaging for vesicoureteral reflux–is there a better way? J Urol 174:7–8.

9. Thompson M, Simon SD, Sharma V, Alon US (2005) Timing of follow-up voiding cystourethrogram in children with primary vesicoureteral reflux: development and application of a clinical algorithm. Pediatrics 115:426–34.

10. Stein R, Thuroff JW (2004) Correction of vesicoureteral reflux: where do we stand? Curr Opin Urol 14:219–225.

11. Aaronson IA (2005) Does deflux alter the paradigm for the management of children with vesicoureteral reflux? Curr Urol Rep 6:152–156.

12. No authors listed (1981) Medical versus surgical treatment of primary vesicoureteral reflux: a prospective international reflux study in children. J Urol 125:277–283.

13. Edwards D, Normand IC, Prescod N, Smellie JM (1977) Disappearance of vesicoureteric reflux during long-term prophylaxis of urinary tract infection in children. Br Med J 2:285–288.

14. Smellie JM, Normand C (1979) Reflux nephropathy in childhood. In: Hodson CJ, Kincaid-Smith P (eds) Reflux nephropathy. Masson Publishing USA, New York, pp 14–20.

15. Bellinger MF, Duckett JW (1984) Vesicoureteral reflux: a comparison of non-surgical and surgical management. Contrib Nephrol 39:81–93.

16. Arant BS, Jr. Medical management of mild and moderate vesicoureteral reflux: followup studies of infants and young children. A preliminary report of the Southwest Pediatric Nephrology Study Group. J Urol 1992; 148(5 Pt 2):1683–7.

17. Skoog SJ, Belman AB, Majd M (1987) A nonsurgical approach to the management of primary vesicoureteral reflux. J Urol 138:941–946.

18. Goldraich NP, Goldraich IH (1992) Followup of conservatively treated children with high and low grade vesicoureteral reflux: a prospective study. J Urol 148:1688–1692.

19. Duckett JW (1983) Vesicoureteral reflux: a 'conservative' analysis. Am J Kidney Dis 3:139–144.

20. McLorie GA, McKenna PH, Jumper BM, Churchill BM, Gilmour RF, Khoury AE (1990) High grade vesicoureteral reflux: analysis of observational therapy. J Urol 1990; 144:537–540; discussion 545.

21. Weiss R, Tamminen-Mobius T, Koskimies O et al (1992) Characteristics at entry of children with severe primary vesicoureteral reflux recruited for a multicenter, international therapeutic trial comparing medical and surgical management. The International Reflux Study in Children. J Urol 1992; 148:1644–1649.

22. Weiss R, Duckett J, Spitzer A (1992) Results of a randomized clinical trial of medical versus surgical management of infants and children with grades III and IV primary vesicoureteral reflux (United States). The International Reflux Study in Children. J Urol 148:1667–1673.

23. Tamminen-Mobius T, Brunier E, Ebel KD et al (1992) Cessation of vesicoureteral reflux for 5 years in infants and children allocated to medical treatment. The International Reflux Study in Children. J Urol 148:1662–1666.

24. Politano VA, Leadbetter WF (1958) An operative technique for the correction of vesicoureteral reflux. J Urol 79:932–941.

25. Politano VA (1963) One hundred reimplantations and five years. J Urol 90:696–701.

26. Hendren WH (1968) Ureteral reimplantation in children. J Pediatr Surg 3:649–664.

27. Price SE Jr, Johnson SH 3rd, Marshall M Jr (1970) Experience with ureteral reimplantation in the treatment of recurring urinary infections in childhood. J Urol 103:485–490.

28. Carpentier PJ, Bettink PJ, Hop WC, Schroder FH (1982) Reflux–a retrospective study of 100 ureteric reimplantations by the Politano-Leadbetter method and 100 by the Cohen technique. Br J Urol 54:230–233.
29. Steffens L, Steffens J, Sohn M (1986) Indications and results of Politano-Leadbetter antireflux-plasty in 565 cases of ureterorenal surgery]. Urologe A 25:354–357.
30. Burbige KA (1991) Ureteral reimplantation: a comparison of results with the cross-trigonal and Politano-Leadbetter techniques in 120 patients. J Urol 146:1352–1353.
31. Ellsworth PI, Merguerian PA (1995) Detrusorrhaphy for the repair of vesicoureteral reflux: comparison with the Leadbetter-Politano ureteroneocystostomy. J Pediatr Surg 30:600–603.
32. Cohen SJ (1975) Ureterozystoneostomie. Eine neue antirefluxtechnik. Akt Urol 6:1–8.
33. Ahmed S (1978) Ureteral reimplantation by the transverse advancement technique. J Urol 119:547–550.
34. Ehrlich RM (1982) Success of the transvesical advancement technique for vesicoureteral reflux. J Urol 128:554–557.
35. Wacksman J (1983) Initial results with the Cohen cross-trigonal ureteroneocys-totomy. J Urol 129:1198–1199.
36. Glassberg KI, Laungani G, Wasnick RJ, Waterhouse K (1985) Transverse ureteral advancement technique of ureteroneocystostomy (Cohen reimplant) and a modifi-cation for difficult cases (experience with 121 ureters). J Urol 1985; 134:304–307.
37. McCool AC, Joseph DB (1995) Postoperative hospitalization of children under-going cross-trigonal ureteroneocystostomy. J Urol 154:794–796.
38. Kennelly MJ, Bloom DA, Ritchey ML, Panzl AC (1995) Outcome analysis of bilateral Cohen cross-trigonal ureteroneocystostomy. Urology 46:393–395.
39. Lich R, Howerton LW, Davis LA (1961) Recurrent urosepsis in children. 86:554.
40. Gregoir W, Vanregemorter G. (1964) Congenital vesico-ureteral reflux. Urol Int 18:122–136.
41. McDuffie RW, Litin RB, Blundon KE (1977) Ureteral reimplantation: Lich method. Urology 10:19–22.
42. Hampel N, Richter-Levin D, Gersh I (1977) Extravesical repair of primary vesicoureteral reflux in children. J Urol 117:355–357.
43. Marberger M, Altwein JE, Straub E, Wulff SH, Hohenfellner R (1978) The Lich-Gregoir antireflux plasty: experiences with 371 children. J Urol 120:216–219.
44. Bruskewitz R, Sonneland AM, Waters RF (1979) Extravesical ureteroplasty. J Urol 121:648–649.
45. Arap S, Abrao EG, Menezes de Goes G (1981) Treatment and prevention of complications after extravesical antireflux technique. Eur Urol 7:263–267.
46. Linn R, Ginesin Y, Bolkier M, Levin DR (1989) Lich-Gregoir anti-reflux operation: a surgical experience and 5–20 years of follow-up in 149 ureters. Eur Urol 16: 200–203.
47. Heimbach D, Bruhl P, Mallmann R (1995) Lich-Gregoir anti-reflux procedure; indications and results with 283 vesicoureteral units. Scand J Urol Nephrol 29: 311–316.
48. Daines SL, Hodgson NB (1971) Management of reflux in total duplication anomalies. J Urol 1971; 105:720–724.
49. Zaontz MR, Maizels M, Sugar EC, Firlit CF (1987) Detrusorrhaphy: extravesical ureteral advancement to correct vesicoureteral reflux in children. J Urol 138: 947–949.
50. Wacksman J, Gilbert A, Sheldon CA (1992) Results of the renewed extravesical reimplant for surgical correction of vesicoureteral reflux. J Urol 148:359–361.

51. Houle AM, McLorie GA, Heritz DM, McKenna PH, Churchill BM, Khoury AE (1992) Extravesical nondismembered ureteroplasty with detrusorrhaphy: a renewed technique to correct vesicoureteral reflux in children. J Urol 148:704–707.

52. Burbige KA, Miller M, Connor JP (1996) Extravesical ureteral reimplantation: results in 128 patients. J Urol 155:1721–1722.

53. Matouschek E (1981) New concept for the treatment of vesico-ureteral reflux. Endoscopic application of Teflon. Arch Esp Urol 34:385–388.

54. Geiss S, Alessandrini P, Allouch G et al (1990) Multicenter survey of endoscopic treatment of vesicoureteral reflux in children. Eur Urol 17:328–329.

55. Dewan PA, Goh DW (1994) Subureteric polytef injection in the management of vesico-ureteric reflux in children. J Paediatr Child Health 30:324–327.

56. Merckx L, De Boe V, Braeckman J, Verboven M, Piepsz A, Keuppens F (1995) Endoscopic submucosal Teflon injection (STING): an alternative treatment of vesicoureteric reflux in children. Eur J Pediatr Surg 5:34–36.

57. Puri P (1995) Ten year experience with subureteric Teflon (polytetrafluoroethylene) injection (STING) in the treatment of vesico-ureteric reflux. Br J Urol 75:126–131.

58. Leonard MP, Canning DA, Peters CA, Gearhart JP, Jeffs RD (1991) Endoscopic injection of glutaraldehyde cross-linked bovine dermal collagen for correction of vesicoureteral reflux. J Urol 145:115–119.

59. Frey P, Lutz N, Jenny P, Herzog B (1995) Endoscopic subureteral collagen injection for the treatment of vesicoureteral reflux in infants and children. J Urol 154:804–807.

60. Stenberg A, Lackgren G (1995) A new bioimplant for the endoscopic treatment of vesicoureteral reflux: experimental and short-term clinical results. J Urol 154:800–803.

61. Atala A, Keating MA (2002) Vesicoureteral reflux and megaureter. In: Walsh PC, Retik AB, Vaughan ED Jr, Wein AJ (eds) Campbell's urology, vol 2. W. B. Saunders, Philadelphia, PA, pp 2053–2116.

62. Lackgren G, Wahlin N, Skoldenberg E, Stenberg A (2001) Long-term followup of children treated with dextranomer/hyaluronic acid copolymer for vesicoureteral reflux. J Urol 166:1887–1892.

63. Kershen RT, Fefer SD, Atala A (2000) Tissue-engineered therapies for the treatment of urinary incontinence and vesicoureteral reflux. World J Urol 18:51–55.

64. Reddy PK, Evans RM (1994) Laparoscopic ureteroneocystostomy. J Urol 152:2057–2059.

65. Gill IS, Ponsky LE, Desai M, Kay R, Ross JH (2001) Laparoscopic cross-trigonal Cohen ureteroneocystostomy: novel technique. J Urol 166:1811–1814.

66. McDougall EM, Urban DA, Kerbl K et al (1995) Laparoscopic repair of vesicoureteral reflux utilizing the Lich-Gregoir technique in the pig model. J Urol 153:497–500.

67. Lakshmanan Y, Fung LC (2000) Laparoscopic extravesicular ureteral reimplantation for vesicoureteral reflux: recent technical advances. J Endourol 14:589–593, discussion 593–594.

68. Shu T, Cisek LJ Jr, Moore RG (2004) Laparoscopic extravesical reimplantation for postpubertal vesicoureteral reflux. J Endourol 18:441–446.

69. Olsen LH, Deding D, Yeung CK, Jorgensen TM (2003) Computer assisted laparoscopic pneumovesical ureter reimplantation a.m. Cohen: initial experience in a pig model. APMIS Suppl 2003(109):23–25.

70. Peters CA (2004) Robotically assisted surgery in pediatric urology. Urol Clin North Am 31:743–752.

71. Willi U, Treves S (1983) Radionuclide voiding cystography. Urol Radiol 5: 161–173, 175.
72. Mackie GG, Stephens FD (1975) Duplex kidneys: a correlation of renal dysplasia with position of the ureteral orifice. J Urol 114:274–280.
73. Hulbert WC, Duckett JW (1992) Posterior urethral valve obstruction. American Urological Association Update Series, vol XI, lesson 29, 1992.
74. van Gool JD, Hjalmas K, Tamminen-Mobius T, Olbing H (1992) Historical clues to the complex of dysfunctional voiding, urinary tract infection and vesicoureteral reflux. The International Reflux Study in Children. J Urol 148:1699–1702.
75. Naseer SR, Steinhardt GF (1997) New renal scars in children with urinary tract infections, vesicoureteral reflux and voiding dysfunction: a prospective evaluation. J Urol 158:566–568.

11 Robotic Orchiopexy

Bartley G. Cilento and David Diamond

1. INTRODUCTION

We assume that the readers of this chapter on robotically assisted orchiopexy have familiarly with conventional laparoscopic orchiopexy. Diagnostic laparoscopy and laparoscopy orchiopexy are now well established as safe and effective treatments for the intra-abdominal testis (IAT). However, the use of robotic laparoscopy is new, and the technique still undergoing evaluation as a viable alternative to conventional laparoscopy. The major advantage of the robotic system is to enhance manipulation of tissues, optical magnification, and ease of complex tasks such as suturing. Initially, several types of robotic assistance were available for surgical applications: the da Vinci (Intuitive Surgical, Sunnyvale, CA) and the Zeus (Computer Motion, now Intuitive Surgical, Sunnyvale, CA) systems, with similar basic designs. The two original companies have now merged, and the Zeus system may ultimately be discontinued. The da Vinci system is perhaps the most widely used, and it has early experience in pediatric urologic practice. These robotic systems are expensive and complex to set up and operate. The price of the da Vinci system is in excess of $1 million. The robotic instruments have a limited number of uses (10), and they are relatively expensive. Yearly maintenance contracts for the robotic system, including parts, labor, and replacement of working instruments, approximate $100,000 dollars/year. Extensive training is needed for the operating room staff and to maintain a core of trained personnel. It is expected that costs and efficiency will improve over time, but this is likely dependent of many factors. Nevertheless, these robotic systems have shown a clear advantage in the performance of challenging complex

From: *Current Clinical Urology: Urologic Robotic Surgery*
Edited by: J. A. Stock, M. P. Esposito, and V. J. Lanteri © Humana Press, Totowa, NJ

laparoscopic maneuvers. The precise role of robotics surgery is currently unclear, but it will likely have an advantage in selected applications *(1)*.

The robotic system allows for smooth and natural movements of complex tasks such are suture manipulations and tying. These tasks and all others are aided by a three-dimensional image achieved by a binocular endoscope and a binocular viewing system. In addition, hand actuators are electronically linked and computer processed to control the laparoscopic instruments that have a full 6° of freedom, mimicking the natural movement of the human wrist. Other features include tremor reduction and scale movements. Contrast this with the two-dimensional view of standard laparoscopy and the limited movement of standard laparoscopic instruments, which do not have a full 6° of freedom. Thus, the conventional laparoscopist may need to perform paradoxical movements where the instrument is moved to the right to achieve an internal movement to the left. The limitations of conventional laparoscopy and the required precision of pediatric urologic surgery have hindered the advancement and widespread incorporation of laparoscopy in pediatric urology.

In general, robotic assisted laparoscopy adds a new dimension to laparoscopic surgery, and it is particularly useful for complex tasks such as intracorporeal suturing. Currently, its disadvantages include its high cost, lack of smaller entry ports, and relatively larger instrument sizes *(1)*.

2. LITERATURE REVIEW

PubMed was used to survey the published literature. Fifty-six articles were listed for "laparoscopic orchiopexy" in patients 18 years or younger, but only one article was listed under "robotic laparoscopy" (this article also was captured in the original search). This article described and assessed the feasibility and applicability of using surgeon-controlled robotic arms as a substitute for surgical assistants during urologic laparoscopic surgery *(2)*. Seventeen cases were studied, but only one case was an orchiopexy procedure.

3. SURGICAL ANATOMY

In the majority of boys, the location of the IAT in just proximal to the internal inguinal ring. In rare instances, the testis may be located outside of this proximity. In rare instances, the IAT may have undergone intrauterine torsion, resulting in an intra-abdominal "vanishing" testis (IAVT). In this case, the laparoscopist must identify to his or her satisfaction the confluence of the vas deferens and spermatic vessels to make

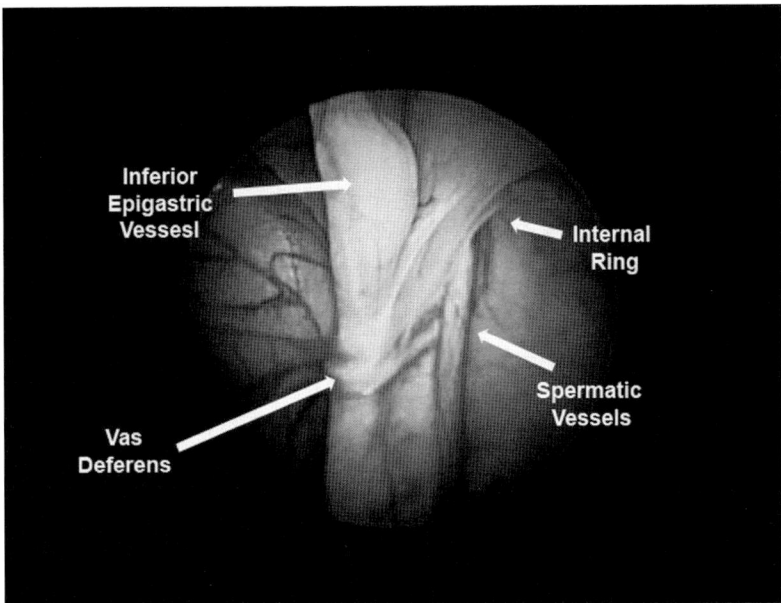

Fig. 1. Laparoscopic view of a normal right internal inguinal ring. The vas deferens and spermatic vessels are labeled. The relationship with the iliac vessels, the inferior epigastric vessels and the obliterated umbilical artery should be familiar to any surgeon evaluating nonpalpable testes laparoscopically.

the diagnosis of a vanished testis. Figure 1 demonstrates the normal anatomy of the inguinal ring with a normally descended testicle. Figure 2 illustrates the anatomy of the internal ring in a boy found to have an IAT.

4. PREOPERATIVE ASSESSMENT

Some healthcare providers attempt to locate the nonpalpable testis with radiologic imaging. The most common modality is ultrasound, but other modalities include magnetic resonance imaging or computed tomography imaging. There is evidence to suggest that these tests are not necessary, insufficiently sensitive, and add undue cost. In nearly all cases, it does not alter the need for surgery or the surgical approach. Just after the induction of anesthesia, the child should be reexamined. Infrequently, a previously nonpalpable testis may become palpable under anesthesia, obviating the need for laparoscopy. There are no additional or

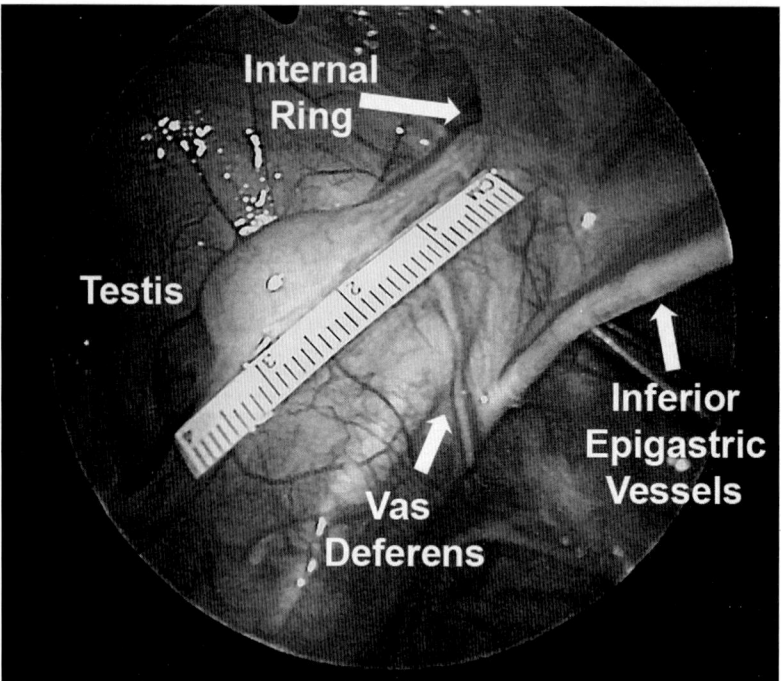

Fig. 2. Laparoscopic view of an IAT. The vas deferens may be seen running from the epididymis over the iliac vessels into the deep pelvis.

specific preoperative studies that are required before performing a robotic orchiopexy. Consideration may be given to establishing blood type in the rare chance that intraoperative transfusion would be necessary secondary to a vascular injury.

5. INSTRUMENTATION

The da Vinci Surgical System is composed of a surgeon console and surgical cart that houses the robotic arms. The surgical cart is positioned at the patient's side with sterile draping. It contains the three working arms with articulating joints to allow full flexibility in positioning. The middle arm holds the binocular endoscope, whereas to two outer arms hold the working laparoscopic instruments. All three arms are controlled from the surgeon's console. The operating surgeon is seated at the console and looks into the three-dimensional visual system. His or her hands are placed into a pair of mobile actuators with full mobility that is replicated by the intracorporeal instruments. There are a variety of grasping and cutting instruments that may be used, and a cautery device. A foot pedal integrated into the surgeon's console activates the cautery device. The endoscope can be manipulated by pressing a foot pedal clutch that transfers control from the working arms to the endoscope arm. A fully scrubbed surgical assistant who observes the surgical procedure from a standard two-dimensional monitor changes instruments. These changes take no longer than conventional laparoscopy once familiarity is achieved. The endoscope and working instruments are placed through the laparoscopic cannulae. The working instruments are 8 mm in diameter, and the endoscope is 12 mm. These dimensions are large by today's pediatric laparoscopy standards, but 5-mm instruments are currently available. A fourth arm system is available to provide static retraction, but it is rarely needed.

6. PATIENT POSITION

The patient is placed in the supine position. The pelvis is slightly elevated by placing a fold blanket or jell pad beneath the buttocks. The bladder is catheterized and decompressed, but an indwelling catheter is not left in place. The stomach is decompressed by passage of a nasogastric or orogastric tube. Two peripheral intravenous catheters are placed for intravascular access. The patient is prepped and draped in the usual sterile manner with the upper boundary being the xiphoid, the lateral boundary the mid-axillary line, and the lower boundary the scrotum and upper thighs.

7. OPERATING ROOM SETUP

With an experience team, set up takes about 20 min, which includes connecting the components (surgical cart, surgeon's console, and satellite monitor), running through the startup sequence, and draping the surgical cart. The specified endoscope (0, 30, or 60° lens in the up or down position) must be in place for the proper calibration sequence to occur. In most cases, the 30° down configuration works best. There is an additional 10 min to complete final positioning of the surgical cart and engage the robot.

8. PORT PLACEMENT

Port placements for a right and bilateral robotic orchiopexy are depicted in Figures 3 and 4. Port placement for a left robotic orchiopexy would be the mirror image of the right robotic orchiopexy. The scrubbed surgeons gain initial intra-abdominal entry by using the Hasson technique

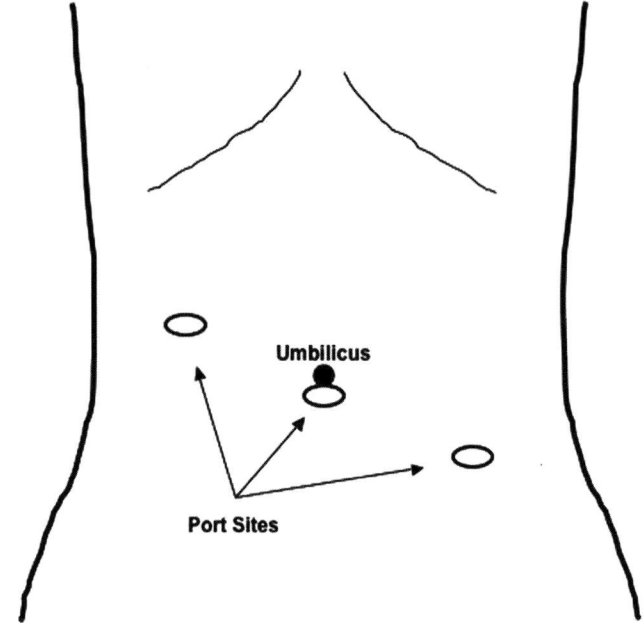

Fig. 3. Port placement for a right IAT.

via an infraumbilical incision. Vicryl sutures (3-0) are place in the abdominal fascia and used to secure the 10-mm cannula once placed. Once the infraumbilical port is placed, the abdomen is insufflated with carbon dioxide to obtain an intra-abdominal pressure of 15 mmHg. The pressure limit should be set at 15 mmHg, but the gas flow setting may be set at 4 to 5 l/min. As gas dissipates through the trocar ports, a flow rate of 4–5 l/min will quickly compensate to maintain an adequate pneumoperitoneum. By hand, the endoscope is introduced through the umbilical port. Under direct vision, the other two 10-mm ports are placed using a trocar/cannula system. The trocars are secured with Vicryl sutures in the same fashion as the umbilical trocar. All three cannulae are specifically designed to dock to the robotic arms. At this point, the robotic arms are "docked" to the cannulae. Using the manual activated clutching mechanism located on the robotic arms, the three arms are placed in the approximate orientation to perform the robotic orchiopexy. The surgeon at the console makes final adjustments remotely, and the robotic orchiopexy can proceed in the same manner as a conventional laparoscopic orchiopexy, which may include a single-stage orchiopexy or a two stage orchiopexy.

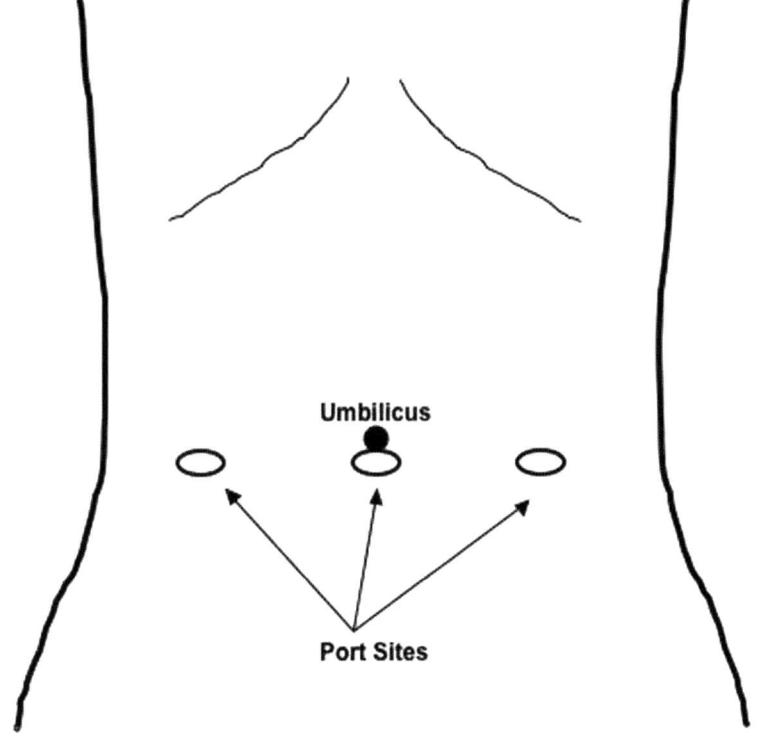

Fig. 4. Port positioning for a bilateral IAT.

9. STEP-BY-STEP APPROACH

Once seated at the console, the operative procedure continues by first sweeping the bowel cephalad. Next, the normal internal inguinal ring of the descended contralateral side is viewed as a reference and to ensure there is no subclinical patent processus vaginalis.

The clinically affected side is examined next. Intrauterine torsion of a descended testes should be suspected when the laparoscopist demonstrates the following: (1) closed internal inguinal ring, (2) vas deferens entering the internal ring, and (3) diminutive spermatic vessels entering the internal inguinal ring. Our preference is to subsequently perform an inguinal exploration to confirm the findings and remove the atrophic testis. On rare occasions, a normal-looking testis has been found, and a standard inguinal orchiopexy is performed. The diagnosis of the IAVT is established when the laparoscopist finds the following: (1) closed internal inguinal ring and (2) vas deferens and spermatic vessels ending blindly together within the abdomen. No further procedures are necessary except to consider contralateral orchiopexy (which is the preference of BC). Although the IAT can be located anywhere from the level of the kidney to the deep pelvis, the majority of the IAT are located within several centimeters of the internal inguinal ring (Fig. 3). Once located, the surgeon must make the decision to perform one of three surgical procedures: (1) a two-stage laparoscopic orchiopexy (Fowler–Stephens technique), (2) a single-stage laparoscopic orchiopexy with preservation of the spermatic vessels, or (3) a single-stage Fowler–Stephens orchiopexy. The least desirable option is the single-stage Fowler–Stephens technique due to a higher incidence of subsequent testicular atrophy. Currently, our preferred method is the two-stage laparoscopic Fowler–Stephens technique. The first and second stages are separated by 4 to 6 months. During the first stage, the diagnosis of IAT is established, and the spermatic vessels are ligated by placement of surgical clips. Two surgical clips are placed proximally and one clip is placed distally. This is accomplished by grasping the spermatic vessels without any attempt to dissect the posterior peritoneum and create a "window" under the spermatic vessels. Unnecessary dissection results in scar formation, which can make the second procedure more difficult. The second procedure is scheduled 4–6 months later to allow for hypertrophy of the deferential vessels, which will now be the primary blood supply to the testis once the second stage is completed. Although there is theoretically, a third blood supply via the cremasteric vessels, it is hard to reliably identify and preserve. Therefore, it cannot be relied upon after completion of the second stage, because it may be disrupted during the second stage dissection and mobilization.

As can be viewed in the accompanying video, the spermatic vessels are transected, which allows for better manipulation of the testis and facilitates further dissection of the posterior peritoneum, which contains the vas deferens, deferential artery, and any accompanying collateral vasculature. The second maneuver is to transect the gubernaculum. This is best done by sequential retraction of the gubernaculum to ensure that the distal extent of the gubernaculum is visualized and transected. This step is advisable to help reduce inadvertent injury to a long looping vas deferens, which may or may not be recognized or discernible. Mobilization of the testicle continues by incising the lateral aspect of the posterior peritoneum. The intra-abdominal testis is largely free at this point with its blood supply coming from the deferential artery contained with the medially based peritoneal "pedicle." If further mobilization is needed, the medially based peritoneal pedicle can be reflected off the iliac vessels. This is generally an easy dissection. At this point, the laparoscopist should deliberately identify the ureter and vas deferens to prevention injury to either structure.

The procedure continues by creation of a peritoneal window medial to the obliterated umbilical ligament but lateral to the bladder. Be sure to make the window sufficiently large to facilitate passage of the testicle through this opening. Consideration can be given to partial development and dissection of the tunnel beyond the peritoneal opening. This maneuver is not always necessary. At this point, the intracorporeal surgery is halted while the scrotal incision and creation of the subdartos pouch is performed. Establishment of intra-abdominal access from the scrotum can be achieved in several ways. A reusable 5-mm trocar can be back loaded over a 3- or 5-mm laparoscopic instrument, which is advanced into the abdomen under direct vision. Once the tip of the laparoscopic instrument appears through the peritoneal window, the 5-mm trocar is advanced along the shaft of the instrument into the abdomen. Alternatively, a 5- or 10-mm radially dilating sheath (as used commonly used for peritoneal access via the Veress technique) can be passed from the scrotal incision through the peritoneal window under direct vision. Once intra-abdominal access is achieved via the scrotum, a laparoscopic grasper is placed through the scrotal port, and the testis is grasped. The orientation of the testicle and peritoneal pedicle is checked to avoid twisting of the peritoneal pedicle and blood supply. The testis is then pulled through the peritoneal window into the scrotum. We have found it helpful to use Ragnell retractors to separate the scrotal incision and subsequently grasp the gubernaculum with a hemostat as it appears. There is commonly resistance of the testis as it passes thru the newly created canal. Slow continual traction, a rocking back and forth, and dilation of the canal with the Ragnell retractors are all maneuvers that can help aid the passage of the testicle. Once the testicle is within the scrotum, the orchiopexy can proceed as customary. Surgeon preferences vary regarding the ways to perform scrotal fixation of the testis, and some surgeons do not perform scrotal fixation. The scrotal skin is closed with a rapidly absorbing suture in either a running or interrupted manner.

The abdomen is surveyed for any evidence of bleeding. The trocars are sequentially removed under direct vision. The fascial edges at the port entry sites are closed with interrupted absorbable sutures. The abdominal fascia at the port entry sites are infiltrated with 0.25% Marcaine as well as the skin edges. Subcuticular interrupted deep dermal sutures using Monocryl suture reapproximate the skin edges. A skin sealant is applied to the scrotum, and a dressing is applied over the port sites.

In general, this procedure is performed on an outpatient basis, and postoperative discomfort is managed with acetaminophen with or without codeine.

10. SPECIAL CONSIDERATIONS

There is no data on the operative success of the robotic laparoscopic orchiopexy. Theoretically, the results should not differ significantly from conventional laparoscopy, but this remains to be proven. It has been reported that the incidence of testicular atrophy after laparoscopic orchiopexy varies by the surgical approached used: 2% for single-stage orchiopexy, 22% for one-stage Fowler–Stephens, and 10% for two-stage Fowler–Stephens (3). The advantages of the robotic surgical system are the ease in which complex laparoscopic maneuvers can be performed and increased optical magnification. Nevertheless, there is a physical disassociation of the surgeon with the patient and operative field. This requires is a great reliance on the skill and attentiveness other members of the surgical team for the procedure to progress smoothly, efficiently, and safely. Without question, the robotic orchiopexy imparts significantly greater cost, whereas the postoperative advantages over conventional laparoscopy have yet to be proven.

11. MANAGEMENT OF COMPLICATIONS

The most significant complication is vascular injury, which usually occurs during trocar placement. Small vessel injury that might involve mesenteric vessels can be handled with cautery; however, large vessel injury results in an emergent laparotomy, control of the bleeding, intravascular volume repletion, and emergent consultation with a vascular surgeon. Bowel injury may occur during intra-abdominal access or possibly a thermal injury during intracorporeal dissection. The degree of injury will dictate the response. Superficial or minor thermal contact with the bowel can often be managed expectantly. More significantly thermal injury or lacerations should prompt a consultation with a general surgeon. Bladder puncture occurring during initial intra-abdominal access can be avoided with bladder decompression. Herniation of intra-abdominal contents through the fascial ports sites can be avoided by fascial closure. Finally, atrophy of the testicle after orchiopexy is handled by expectant management, and it does not require orchiectomy.

REFERENCES

1. Cilento BG, Peters CP (2004) Laparoscopic and robotic surgery in pediatric urology. Atlas Urol Clin 12:143–157.
2. Partin AW, Adams JB, Moore RG, Kavoussi LR (1995) Complete robot-assisted laparoscopic urologic surgery: a preliminary report. J Am Coll Surg 181:552–557.
3. Baker LA, Docimo SG, Surer I, et al (2001) A multi-institutional analysis of laparoscopic orchiopexy. BJU Int 87:484–489.

IV OTHER CONSIDERATIONS FOR ROBOTIC SURGERY

12   Robotic Suturing

Scott J. Belsley and Garth H. Ballantyne

1. INTRODUCTION

Fundamentals of proper surgical suturing require an opposition of tissue planes in a manner that facilitates healing while limiting the inflammatory response and damage to surrounding tissue. Hypothetical benefits of telerobotic surgery over traditional minimally invasive instrumentation are provided through tremor filtration, motion scaling, articulation, and improved ergonomics. Although surgical suturing seems like a natural application of the increased intracorporeal dexterity afforded by this refined technology, there are a multitude of factors involved that obfuscate such an apparent revelation.

The placement of sutures to oppose tissue planes depends on several factors. These factors are dependent not only on a surgeon's technical abilities but also on a multitude of variables ranging from medical comorbidities to operating room staffing. We present a background in basic technique and a review of individual studies to suggest a context for the evolution of robotic suturing.

2. METHODOLOGY

A systems approach and component evaluation of the steps necessary to telerobotically oppose tissue planes are merited. Critical studies of surgical systems such as laparoscopy, robots, or virtual reality simulators that inherently evaluate the kinematics and dynamics of the steps of the procedure benefit from a regimented methodology for both analysis of efficacy and objective evaluation *(1)*.

This systems approach is beneficial not only for the individual steps in knot tying or port placement but also for the entire design of the operating room and the rolls of the individuals participating in the operating room

From: *Current Clinical Urology: Urologic Robotic Surgery*
Edited by: J. A. Stock, M. P. Esposito, and V. J. Lanteri © Humana Press, Totowa, NJ

suite. Thus, the proper design of the entire operating room experience is critical in minimally invasive surgery so that surgeons may dedicate their physical and mental energy toward the technical and anatomic challenges of the operation instead of the mechanics of the instrumentation (2). Not only can the physical efficiency of the individual actions behind minimally invasive suturing be improved by such an approach (3) but also, in a more global context, minimally invasive surgery is performed more efficiently in a dedicated surgical suite versus a traditional operating room (4).

3. THEORY AND HISTORY

Surgical techniques of suturing share similar goals: creation of an anastomosis safely, rapidly, and efficiently. An ideal technique limits the amount of intramural foreign body and tissue trauma, with the expectation of a decreased inflammatory response. Ideal results achieve rapid and substantial healing in a systemic manner that minimizes intersurgeon variability.

Paramount to the description of surgical anastomosis was Lembert's treatise that serosa-to-serosa approximation was necessary to provide early adhesion formation and subsequent permanent anastomotic strength (5). Shortly thereafter, Halstead (6) demonstrated that it is actually the submucosal layer and not the serosa that is responsible for the strength and integrity of the intestines.

Although anatomic layers vary between tissues, coaptation of wound surfaces is necessary to provide conditions for primary wound healing. Sutures, however, are foreign bodies with potentially negative effects on the healing process (7,8). Inflammatory reaction in a wound is caused not only by direct injury to the tissue but also by foreign material present in the wound area. This inflammatory reaction in the wound region is exaggerated directly by an increase number of passages of needles and sutures and indirectly with the presence of excess suture material. Brunius (9) confirmed these findings and demonstrated a prolongation of the inflammatory reaction when sutures were used.

The adage of "do no harm" holds true to surgical suturing. Sutures should be used to approximate tissue planes so that the body's natural mechanisms for healing are least disrupted. Sutures placed by hand through the wall of the gut produce local inflammation at the anastomosis regardless of the type of suture, because it is the penetration of the suture through the bowel layers that initiates this response (10).

There have been many different technologies developed to aid in surgical anastomosis over the past 100 years. Denans' rings used two solid rings of identical dimensions, placed inside of each end of transected intestine and joined together by an expanding cylinder coil *(11)*. This device was followed by the Murphy button, which consisted of two hemispheric ends placed inside the bowel and screwed together to form the anastomosis *(12)*. Surgical staplers were introduced by the Hungarian surgeon Hultl in 1908 *(13)*. Surgeons in the former Soviet Union initially applied the idea for pulmonary resections in tuberculosis hospitals and later for gastric surgery. These devices were introduced into the United States by Ravitch in the 1960s, and since that time they have been achieving increasing popularity *(14)*.

4. ERGONOMICS

Laparoscopic suturing is limited by the design of the instrumentation compounded by small working spaces and fixed angles at the trocar level to place sutures. A comparison of the physical effort required for laparo-scopic and open surgery has been quantitated. These studies indicate that a minimally invasive surgeon must use both increased physical and cognitive work to overcome the separation between the surgeon and the operating field. In comparison with open surgery where the surgeon views and manipulates patient's tissues directly and naturally by using simple and efficient instruments, the laparoscopic surgeon must view the operating field indirectly through an optical and video system and simul-taneously manipulate tissues by using more complex and less efficient instruments. Under these conditions, the laparoscopic surgeon has to work harder from the very beginning to achieve the same technical goals as those of open surgery *(15)*.

A typical disposable laparoscopic grasper transmits the force of the surgeon's hand from the handle to the tip with a ratio of only 1:3 in contrast to a 3:1 ratio with a hemostat *(16)*. The surgeon must therefore work about 6 times as hard to accomplish the same grasping task with the laparoscopic instrument *(17)*. Excessive wrist angulation, whether flexion/extension or radial/ulnar deviation, decreases the efficiency of the forearm muscle actuating the hand and fingers and increases carpal tunnel pressure *(18,19)*.

Electromyographic signals and body part discomfort scores are higher during laparoscopic knot tying versus their open correlate. Complex manipulative tasks using laparoscopic techniques require substantially higher upper extremity muscle effort compared with open surgical techniques *(20)*.

Three categories of hand and wrist problems are typically described, usually occurring after a prolonged high grasping force has been applied to an instrument. These problems include compression neuropathies and pressure injuries to the soft tissues of the hands and fingers, wrist pain, and hand fatigue. Typically, the surgeon might recollect a vague discomfort during the procedure but later describe numbness and pain in the distribution of the digital nerves. The results of long-term injury on laparoscopic surgeons are largely unknown.

A series of studies largely with retrospective questionnaire have evaluated neuromuscular complaints in minimally invasive surgeons. Hand-assisted laparoscopy is associated with more frequent neuromuscular strain to the upper extremity than standard laparoscopy, but standard laparoscopic surgeons experience more neck pain or injury *(21)*. Case reports of laparoscopic tubal anastomosis repeatedly are associated with surgeon fatigue, neck, shoulder, and back pain. Surgeons in these small case studies who compare the procedures to robotic-assisted operations typically describe the later as more comfortable and generating less physical fatigue *(22,23)*. This point has also been made in the description of thoracic robotic procedures *(24)*.

5. COGNITIVE BENEFITS OF ROBOTIC SUTURING

Minimally invasive intracorporeal suturing is a stressful task. Compounding the stress of this technical challenge are the significant cognitive challenges for the laparoscopic surgeon who must overcome the physical separation of the visual and physical aspects of the operation. The surgeons must "blend" or bring together the view on the display and the mechanical feedback from the arms and hands to dexterously manipulate the tissues. A definite cognitive expenditure is involved with reconstructing the three-dimensional (3D) workspace from the two-dimensional (2D) television screen.

Although the use of performance efficiency measures (e.g., speed, movement economy, and errors) and ergonomic assessments are relatively well established, the evaluation of cognitive outcomes is rare. Assessment strategies that include mental workload measures act as a way to improve training scenarios and training/operating environments. These mental workload measures can be crucially important in determining the difference between well-intentioned but subtly distracting technologies and true breakthroughs that will enhance performance and reduce stress *(25)*.

The visual and physical interfaces involved with laparoscopic knot tying have been shown to cause greater stress levels in surgeons as measured by tonic skin conductance level, electrooculogram measuring number of blinks, and subjective reports of stress *(15)*.

Robotics with its comfortable console and intuitive interface decreases the stress of complicated procedures. Participants with no experience as primary surgeons in endoscopic surgery performed a set of simulated surgical tasks by using robotics and a traditional manual endoscopic surgery system. Given identical tasks, the time to completion was longer using the telerobotic technique than its manual counterpart. Despite the increased operative time, a questionnaire measuring the participants' intuitiveness and mental stress and the upper extremity postural analysis suggested that telerobotic surgery provided a more comfortable environment for the surgeon without any additional mental stress *(26)*.

Exact quantification of decreased stress is difficult to substantiate especially considering the confounding factor of the learning curve involved with the new technology and the systems involved. Berguer, however, evaluated electromyographic data, skin conductance, and perceived difficulty to measure both laparoscopic novices and experts performing bench tasks. Robotic techniques seem slower and less precise than laparoscopic technique for simple tasks, but equally fast and possibly less stressful for complex tasks. His studies also suggested that previous laparoscopic experience has a complex influence on the physical and mental adaptation to robotic surgery *(27)*.

The operating room environment no doubt also compounds the influence of experience. Kolvenbach reports a series of minimally invasive aneurysm repairs by using traditional laparoscopic instrumentation and robotic-assisted operations. The time to suture the aortic anastomosis was significantly shorter in the robotic-assistance group, yet total operating time was longer because of the technical complexity of the robotic device *(28)*. Although mental stresses of the operating room environment are present for laparoscopic and robotic procedures, an operating room team that is not yet comfortable with robotic procedures also may increase the stress of the robotic operator.

6. 3D VISUALIZATION AS IT APPLIES TO SURGICAL SUTURING

Stereoscopic vision provides a significant advantage when table drills of increasing complexity are performed with the robotic system in 3D mode compared with 2D mode *(29,30)*. Suturing skill sets evaluated with table anastomosis drills also demonstrate this pattern with anastomosis completed 65% faster using 3D with equal, if not greater, accuracy *(31)*.

More complicated evaluations have been performed comparing motion path analysis of robotic surgery compared with laparoscopy. Moorthy et al. *(32)* and the team at St Mary's Hospital in London used the da

Vinci Application Programming Interface (API) for motion path analysis of positional data to demonstrate enhanced dexterity reduction in terms of path traveled by nearly 50% compared with laparoscopic surgery. 3D vision enhanced measures of dexterity by a further 10–15%. The presence of 3D vision results in a 93% reduction in skills-based errors, and it was required for the robotic operators to have a significant reduction in time taken compared with their laparoscopic cohort *(32)*.

7. NARROW WORKING VIEW AND SUTURE MANIPULATION

The greater magnification and improved optics of the da Vinci Surgical System (Intuitive Surgical, Sunnyvale, CA) also contribute to some problems with suturing for both inexperienced and expert users. Although there are few systemic analyses of novice intracorporeal robotic anastomoses versus laparoscopic anastomoses, the greater magnification sometimes predisposes novel robotic users to place a greater number of sutures per unit length than what is traditionally done with the laparoscopic anastomosis.

A problem that is a function of working in a small workspace is the increased manipulation of the length of the suture material. Although the manipulation of the needle is made easier, the manipulation of the suture itself is more difficult. When working in a narrow field of view, it is often necessary to zoom out of the visual field of the anastomosis to track the motion of the robotic instruments as the slack in the suture is tightened.

Another difficulty with working with suture material in both laparoscopy and robotics lies within the problems with grasping the suture material. Some materials, especially proline, do not have a strong transverse fracture strength. Therefore, when the robotic graspers are used to pull up on the suture and draw out the remaining length of the suture, it requires applying force without haptic feedback to grip the suture material. The weakening of the suture can lead to another cause of possible suture disruption. After infliction of controlled damage with laparoscopic needle holders, sutures of various materials had significantly reduced tensile strength and impaired extension compared with control sutures *(33)*.

The passage of a suture into the operating field is also more difficult with robotic procedures. The 8-mm intuitive ports do not accommodate most curved needles and an additional working port is needed. Although the robotic exterior arms can be removed out of position, this is notably more difficult than laparoscopy where such an action does not necessitate any more of an increase work than a standard instrument change.

A novel idea, which has recently been introduced, is the concept of modified suture design specific for intracorporeal minimally invasive suturing and knot tying. A modified suture allowed inexperienced surgical residents to perform intracorporeal laparoscopic knot tying on average faster than the standard suture. The concept of modifying suture design to facilitate intracorporeal laparoscopic suturing and knot tying will most likely receive further attention *(34)*.

8. HAPTIC FEEDBACK

The application of robotic end wrist technology aids certain characteristics of surgical suture placement. The increased number of degrees of freedom facilitates complex motion tasks and in the execution of more natural circular wristed movements. Although this technology facilitates the task of following the arc of the needle as it passes through various tissues, the lack of haptic feedback implies a difficulty in judging the consistency of the tissue that has been encompassed by the arc of the needle. Additional difficulties arise because it is difficult to gauge the tension that is placed on each stitch causing both suture line tension and the tissue tension (i.e., the surgical adage of "approximation and not strangulation") to rely on visual cues only. This difficulty also is found in surgical knot tying, which is especially problematic, because a perfectly sutured running anastomosis can be rendered incompetent with a loose knot.

End-to-end anastomoses on postmortem porcine small intestine were evaluated by experienced endoscopic surgeons who used either standard endoscopic techniques, robotic assistance, or both. Anastomosis time, number of stitches, and the number of knots did not differ significantly between the two groups. The time needed per stitch was significantly shorter with robot assistance. More suture ruptures occurred, however, in the robot group due to the lack of force feedback. Total anastomosis time was similar for the two groups, but fewer stitch errors were found in the robotic group *(35)*.

Preliminary studies describe evidence that haptic feedback, in the form of sensory substitution, permits the surgeon to apply more consistent, precise, and greater tension to fine suture materials without breakage during robot-assisted knot tying *(35,36)*.

This is not to say that haptic feedback is a prerequisite for surgical suturing but rather that certain caveats must be reinforced. Gentleness in handling tissues is mandatory in closing contaminated wounds. Sutures tied tightly around wound edges markedly increase the incidence of wound infection because of the strangulation of tissue within the suture loop and its associated lowering of the hosts' defenses.

9. MICROSURGICAL ANASTOMOSES AND TREMOR FILTRATION

Microsurgery typically uses 7-0 to 10-0 sutures, which are too small to be seen by the naked eye. The fragility of these sutures also implies that reliance on haptic feedback, even during traditional open procedures, is minimized. With increased visualization, scaling of movements, and the benefits of tremor filtration, microsurgery seems an ideal application for robotic surgery. Studies typically demonstrate that minimally invasive robotic micro-anastomoses are feasible but that no increased patient benefit is accrued compared to the open procedure. Studies typically are limited to the endpoint of an intact anastomosis that can withstand a saline infusion test and that do not evaluate a more holistic view of minimally invasive versus open surgery.

The Zeus robot was used to compare end-to-end microvascular anastomoses in 1-mm rat femoral arteries with interrupted 10-0 suture *(37)*. The study describes the robotic tremor filtration as remarkable. Nonetheless, all hand-sewn anastomoses were patent, none leaked and they were accomplished more rapidly (hand-sewn anastomotic time 17.2 min) than Zeus anastomoses (27.6 min; $p < 0.01$). Consequently, there was no measurable benefit from the tremor filtration and motion scaling offered by robot-enhanced surgery *(37)*.

Kuang et al. *(38)* evaluated the technically difficult vasovasotomy performed with 9-0 sutures by using either the conventional microscope or the robot. Prespecified performance measures and adverse haptic events (e.g., broken sutures, bent needles, or loose stitches) were recorded. Patency was evaluated by instilling saline through the anastomoses. Mean operating time differed significantly (84 vs. 38 min; $p = 0.01$), and numbers of adverse haptic events were higher for robot-assisted vasovasotomy than for microscope-assisted vasovasotomy (84 vs. 38 min, $p = 0.01$; 2.4 vs. 0.0 events, $p = 0.03$). The number of needle passes required for the six full-thickness stitches was similar in both groups (16.8 vs. 15.2 passes; $p = 0.55$). All anastomosis were evaluated by instilling saline and demonstrated to be patent. These authors also remarked about the noticeable elimination of tremor and commented about the use of the robot as a surgical alternative for microsurgical vasovasostomy *(38)*.

These studies are particularly relevant because they demonstrate that robotics is feasible for the even most delicate anastomoses. Of note is that the comparison has changed. Because these procedures are impossible with traditional laparoscopic graspers, robotics is no longer compared with laparoscopy but rather to the open operations.

10. LEARNING CURVES

Considerable training is necessary to master laparoscopic suturing and knot-tying. These difficult skills contribute to reasons why advanced laparoscopic procedures have been met with a certain degree of reluctance. On initial examination, robotic systems are assumed to facilitate these difficult skills, with a steeper learning curve that requires less time to master. This assumption is not always supported by laboratory data. Consistent conclusions are difficult to surmise considering the variety of different drill sets that are used to investigate subtle changes in groups of novices and experts with varying levels of experience.

Robotic suturing in an *ex vivo* bench test is quickly learned. Hernandez et al. *(39)* demonstrated a very efficient learning curve for the novices by using the da Vinci Surgical System for a series of synthetic small bowel anastomoses. Quantitative analysis used API software to retrieve real-time robotic signal data of time, pathlength, and number of movements. Comparing the first to the fifth anastomosis, the fifth anastomosis took considerably less time (3,507 vs. 2,287 s; $p < 0.01$), fewer total number of movements (2,411 vs. 1,387; $p = 0.01$), and a shorter total pathlength (21,630 vs. 13,941 cm; $p = 0.01$).

Anderson–Hynes pyeloroplasty and Fengerplasty performed with the da Vinci robotic system resulted in overall decreased operative time compared with laparoscopic pyeloroplasty. Factors responsible for the decreased operative time, however, were not clearly defined *(40)*.

Yohannes et al. *(41)* undertook a series of bench trials to evaluate the differences in learning curves between laparoscopy and robotics. Both groups demonstrated a statistically significant improvement between the first and last trial. There were some differences in the laparoscopic learning curves in favor of robotic assistance, however, not for overall improvements.

Conversely, a study compared an *ex vivo* vascular anastomosis using either manual laparoscopic techniques or the Zeus-Aesop system. Similar results were observed for both groups but with significantly longer suture and knot-tying times for the robotic anastomoses. Significantly more actions were needed with the robotic system compared with the manual laparoscopic procedures *(42)*. These *ex vivo* results are both dependent on the task evaluated and operator experience.

Nio et al. *(42,43)* tested a laparoscopically experienced surgeon against a laparoscopically inexperienced surgeon, making alternating laparoscopic vascular anastomoses and robot-assisted laparoscopic vascular anastomoses. The learning curves of both surgeons were not improved by the robotic system. Neither laparoscopic method influenced the quality score or leakage rate, but with laparoscopic experience, significantly fewer failures were made. Suturing and knot tying were faster with laparoscopic experience both with and without the robotic system, and fewer stitch actions and knot actions were performed. Bergeurs' studies *(27)* also suggested that previous laparoscopic experience has a complex influence on the physical and mental adaptation to robotic surgery.

Although studies seem to suggest equivalency between the two techniques, the comparison between learning curves still remains difficult. Laparoscopic suturing is challenging when port placement or visualization is compromised. This is not the case when evaluating an *ex vivo* learning skills task. Early *ex vivo* studies (i.e., performing peg-board tasks) demonstrated that laparoscopic maneuvering and suturing are faster and just as precise when performed manually as when performed with the prototype robotic system, with differences in speed inversely proportional to the size of the suture *(22)*. These findings might represent an investigator-derived task that is particularly well suited to laparoscopy, harkening the need for a regimented skill set as evaluations of surgical skill and new technologies become more common.

11. FUTURE APPLICATION

A glimpse into the future of robotic suturing is perhaps heralded by a short reflection on past developments. The tenants of surgical suturing are based on atraumatic opposition of tissue in a manner that achieves rapid healing and minimizes inflammatory response and inter-surgeon variability. An examination of future suturing applications needs to acquiesce that all these criteria are better met with surgical stapling devices that share both an decreased inflammatory response and accelerated wound healing *(10)*.

The difficulties of using the robotic devices outweighed many of the proposed benefits of tremor filtration and scaling of motions in early attempts at complex microanastomotic procedures. The increases in cardiopulmonary bypass time have limited the acceptance of robotic totally endoscopic coronary artery bypass grafting and complex vascular repairs requiring aortic cross-clamp *(28)*. Although coronary artery and valve suturing initially seemed like ideal applications, time limits are causing surgeons to move away from the suturing abilities of the robot in favor of other facilitating technologies such as the use of nitinol U-clips for mitral valve repairs *(44)* and in favor of anastomotic coupling devices to facilitate beating heart totally endoscopic coronary artery bypass grafting *(41)*. Again, it is important to note that minimally invasive suturing was deemed impossible before the introduction of robotics.

The technical superiority of the robotic device over laparoscopic suturing is evident in complex microanastomoses where laparoscopic approaches are not tenable and the robot seems to at least be equivalent to the open microsurgical approaches. In the near future, robotic suturing will play an invaluable role in urologic and gynecologic procedures that need minimally invasive microanastomoses in the narrow confines of the bony pelvis and that are not limited by the same time constraints as cardiac surgery. Eventually, robotics also will be applied to endoscopic suturing, which is already being studied with histologic evaluation of suture depth placement *(45)* and automated devices to facilitate suture placement and knot tying *(46)*.

In the distant future, telerobotic master-slave devices will evolve into "true" surgical robots. API data that are currently being gathered from research groups performing methodological component evaluation of surgical suturing will be used to increasingly automate the suturing process and eventually entire surgical procedures. There will be a time when the robot performs the surgery with surgeon playing a supervisory role *(1)*.

12. CONCLUSIONS

There is considerable overlap with the number of surgeons who regularly perform complex laparoscopic and robotic procedures that require intracorporeal suturing. Robotics is still in its infancy, and although the technology is indeed "intuitive," the machines are currently being used only by centers that can afford them. It is rare that surgeons, other than urologists, who do not have advanced laparoscopic training perform robotic operations. Long-term prospective follow-up of procedures performed with or without the da Vinci robotic system for surgeons with limited experience in laparoscopic management will help delineate the true efficacy of the device. This will prove particularly true for urological procedures such as radical prostatectomy in which difficult maneuvers are performed using robotic systems. Perhaps with concurrent development of medical advances and facilitating technologies such as visual overlays there will be a physiologic reason to demand increased minimally invasive precision.

Tasks that are easy to perform with traditional laparoscopic instrumentation are not improved with robotic instrumentation. Learning curves for simple *ex vivo* tasks are not improved for novices, and a machine that promises increased precision does not necessarily correlate with improved clinical outcomes. Robotic suturing is superior to traditional laparoscopic approaches only by experienced operators in the correct context. Minimally invasive robotic approaches are, however, possible and comparable with open microsurgical anastomoses that traditionally had to be performed with a microscope. Before the adaptation of the device for urologic and gynecologic procedures, the perils of increased cross-clamping times in cardiovascular surgery limited its clinical practicality. The increased use and the exponential growth of urologic robotic procedures are perhaps more indicative of the future of the technology rather than studies that are brief glimpses of the technology in an artificial environment.

REFERENCES

1. Rosen J et al (2003) Minimally invasive surgery task decomposition–etymology of endoscopic suturing. Stud Health Technol Inform 94:295–301.
2. Lai F, Entin E (2005) Integrating surgical robots into the next medical toolkit. Stud Health Technol Inform 119:285–287.
3. Neo EL, Patkin M, Watson DI (2004) Suturing efficiency during hiatal repair for laparoscopic fundoplication. ANZ J Surg 74:13–17.
4. Hsiao KC, Machaidze Z, Pattaras JG (2004) Time management in the operating room: an analysis of the dedicated minimally invasive surgery suite. JSLS 8: 300–303.
5. Lembert A (1826) Nouveau procede d'enterorraphie. Repertoire. Gen. Anat. Physiol. Pathol. 2:3.
6. Halsted W (1887) Circular suture of the intestine-an experimental study. Am J Med Sci 94:436–461.
7. Postlethwait RW, Willigan DA, Ulin AW (1975) Human tissue reaction to sutures. Ann Surg 181:144–150.
8. Van Winkle W Jr, Hastings JC (1972) Considerations in the choice of suture material for various tissues. Surg Gynecol Obstet 135:113–126.
9. Brunius U, Zederfeldt B, Ahren C (1967) Healing of skin incisions closed by non-suture technique. A tensiometric and histologic study in the rat. Acta Chir Scand 133:509–516.
10. Ballantyne GH (1984) The experimental basis of intestinal suturing. Effect of surgical technique, inflammation, and infection on enteric wound healing. Dis Colon Rectum 27:61–71.
11. Denans FN (1827) Nouveau procede pour la guerision des plaies des intestins. Recueil Soc R Med Marseille 127–131.
12. Murphy J (1892) Cholecysto-intestinal, gastro-intestinal anastomosis and approximation without sutures. Med Rec 42:335–337.
13. Ravitch M, Steichen F, Welter R (1991) Current practice of surgical stapling. Lea & Febiger, Philadelphia, Pennslyvania.
14. Gritsman JJ (1966) Mechanical suture by Soviet apparatus in gastric resection: use in 4,000 operations. Surgery 59:663–669.
15. Berguer R, Smith WD, Chung YH (2001) Performing laparoscopic surgery is significantly more stressful for the surgeon than open surgery. Surg Endosc 15: 1204–1207.
16. Berguer R (1998) Surgical technology and the ergonomics of laparoscopic instruments. Surg Endosc 12:458–462.

17. Berguer R, Forkey DL, Smith WD (2001) The effect of laparoscopic instrument working angle on surgeons' upper extremity workload. Surg Endosc, 15: 1027–1029.

18. Johnson SL (1993) Ergonomic hand tool design. Hand Clin 9:299–311.

19. Winzeler S, Rosenstein BD (1996) Occupational injury and illness of the thumb. Causes and solutions. Aaohn J 44:487–492.

20. Berguer R, Chen J, Smith WD (2003) A comparison of the physical effort required for laparoscopic and open surgical techniques. Arch Surg 138:967–970.

21. Johnston WK 3rd, Hollenbeck BK, Wolf JS Jr (2005) Comparison of neuromuscular injuries to the surgeon during hand-assisted and standard laparoscopic urologic surgery. J Endourol 19:377–381.

22. Margossian H et al (1998) Robotically assisted laparoscopic tubal anastomosis in a porcine model: a pilot study. J Laparoendosc Adv Surg Tech A 8:69–73.

23. Falcone T et al (1999) Full robotic assistance for laparoscopic tubal anastomosis: a case report. J Laparoendosc Adv Surg Tech A 9:107–113.

24. Garcia-Ruiz A et al. (1997) Robotic surgical instruments for dexterity enhancement in thoracoscopic coronary artery bypass graft. J Laparoendosc Adv Surg Tech A 7:277–283.

25. Carswell CM, Clarke D, Seales WB (2005) Assessing mental workload during laparoscopic surgery. Surg Innov 12:80–90.

26. Lee EC et al (2005) Ergonomics and human factors in endoscopic surgery: a comparison of manual vs telerobotic simulation systems. Surg Endosc 19: 1064–1070.

27. Berguer R, Smith W (2005) An ergonomic comparison of robotic and laparoscopic technique: the influence of surgeon experience and task complexity. J Surg Res 134:87–92.

28. Kolvenbach R et al (2004) Total laparoscopically and robotically assisted aortic aneurysm surgery: a critical evaluation. J Vasc Surg 39:771–776.

29. Munz Y et al (2004) The benefits of stereoscopic vision in robotic-assisted performance on bench models. Surg Endosc 18:611–616.

30. Jourdan IC et al (2004) Stereoscopic vision provides a significant advantage for precision robotic laparoscopy. Br J Surg 91:879–885.

31. Badani KK et al (2005) Comparison of two-dimensional and three-dimensional suturing: is there a difference in a robotic surgery setting? J Endourol 19: 1212–1215.

32. Moorthy K et al (2004) Bimodal assessment of laparoscopic suturing skills: construct and concurrent validity. Surg Endosc 18:1608–1612.

33. Bariol SV, Stewart GD, Tolley DA (2005) Laparoscopic suturing: effect of instrument handling on suture strength. J Endourol 19:1127–1133.

34. Tan A, Razvi H (2005) Evaluation of a novel modified suture material designed to facilitate intracorporeal knot tying during laparoscopic surgery. J Endourol 19:1104–1108.

35. Bethea BT et al Application of haptic feedback to robotic surgery. J Laparoendosc Adv Surg Tech A 14:191–195.

36. Kitagawa M et al (2004) Effect of sensory substitution on suture manipulation forces for surgical teleoperation. Stud Health Technol Inform, 2004. 98: p. 157–63.

37. Knight CG et al (2005) Computer-assisted, robot-enhanced open microsurgery in an animal model. J Laparoendosc Adv Surg Tech A 15:182–185.

38. Kuang W et al (2004) Initial evaluation of robotic technology for microsurgical vasovasostomy. J Urol 171:300–303.

39. Hernandez JD et al (2004) Qualitative and quantitative analysis of the learning curve of a simulated surgical task on the da Vinci system. Surg Endosc 18:372–378.

40. Gettman MT et al (2002) A comparison of laparoscopic pyeloplasty performed with the daVinci robotic system versus standard laparoscopic techniques: initial clinical results. Eur Urol 42:453–457, discussion 457–458.

41. Yohannes P et al (2002) Comparison of robotic versus laparoscopic skills: is there a difference in the learning curve? Urology 60:39–45, discussion 45.

42. Nio D et al (2004) The efficacy of robot-assisted versus conventional laparoscopic vascular anastomoses in an experimental model. Eur J Vasc Endovasc Surg 27: 283–286.

43. Nio D et al (2005) Laparoscopic vascular anastomoses: does robotic (Zeus-Aesop) assistance help to overcome the learning curve? Surg Endosc 19:1071–1076.

44. Felger JE et al (2004) Robot-assisted sutureless minimally invasive mitral valve repair. Surg Technol Int 12:185–187.

45. Kleemann M et al (2005) Depth of endoscopically placed sutures: an experimental study in a human cadaver model. Surg Endosc 19:1602–1605.

46. Swain P, Park PO (2004) Endoscopic suturing. Best Pract Res Clin Gastroenterol 18:37–47.

13 Hemostasis

Ayal M. Kaynan

1. INTRODUCTION

Bleeding is war, and there is no turning back. The best way to deal with it is to avoid it in the first place. When bleeding happens, apply direct pressure, expose the important structures, and then cauterize, clip, staple, ligate, or sew. If bleeding is torrential, maintain direct pressure as best as possible and convert to open unflinchingly. The time to anticipate and practice hemostatic maneuvers is now, preferably in a laboratory, because repair of these problems during surgery often requires that it be done correctly the first time lest a small problem avalanche into disaster.

In laparoscopy, effort should be made not to stain the tissues with blood. Even when a mild ooze stops spontaneously, the color change in the field results in several problems. First, the blood needs to be swept or suctioned away to reveal the underlying structures, adding extra work and motion to the surgery. Second, blood causes the surgeon to depend upon memory and imagination to get past the stain and blood to the essential structures. Third, the light becomes increasingly absorbed making it difficult to visualize anything without increasing light intensity. And finally, the laparoscopic suction/irrigators clog easily, as a rule, and changing them with new devices is cumbersome.

2. PREPARATION

Port structure is generally thought of in terms of access to the anatomy of interest; however, the ability to obtain hemostasis also must be considered. At least one 5-/12-mm working port should be placed on every adult case, because it affords introduction of all laparoscopic hemostatic instruments and necessary sutures.

From: *Current Clinical Urology: Urologic Robotic Surgery*
Edited by: J. A. Stock, M. P. Esposito, and V. J. Lanteri © Humana Press, Totowa, NJ

Next, keep a laparoscopic 10-mm (or medium/large) clip applier open on the working table regardless of the plan elected to dissect and control the anatomy. Generally, the 5-mm clips do not hold well for the smaller tissues intended, nor do they disengage well from their appliers. Furthermore, most vessels requiring only a 5-mm clip may be handled easily with virtually any energy source (e.g., bipolar, monopolar, harmonic). As such, only large clips ought to be used. Even pediatric cases are usually best accomplished without the smaller clips—the 5-mm laparoscopic LigaSure suffices, even close to structures intended for preservation. Intuitive Surgical (Sunnyvale, CA) makes a small clip applier as an 8-mm EndoWrist instrument with 100 closures. The inefficiencies of an instrument swap alone do not justify its use; regardless, the assistant should be ready at a moment's notice with a manual laparoscopic clip applier to be used.

If a laparoscopic vascular stapler is used, always have a reload cartridge open on the working table. If the second cartridge is used, a third should be opened automatically, ready to go if needed. Importantly, make certain that the scrub nurse knows how to exchange cartridges efficiently before actually firing the stapler.

A laparoscopic suction/irrigator is essential in any laparoscopic or robotic case. It is an excellent dissection tool: it washes stained tissues, sucks away blood, and may be used to tamponade small bleeders. Do not start until this instrument is in place. Because suction irrigators tend to clog and sometimes need replacement, the tubing should run off the patient separately from all the other cords to prevent much angst in the switch. Many laparoscopists place heparin in the irrigation fluid (5,000 units per liter of normal saline) to prevent clots and clogs, although this author has not found it beneficial.

Have a port closure device such as the Carter-Thomason or Storz fascial closure device, or 2-0 Prolene on a 3-in. straight needle in the room in case of bleeding from deep muscle upon portal access.

Finally, cross-matched blood should be available as appropriate.

3. AVOIDANCE

The form of entry, whether by Hasson or Veress, is generally unimportant on a virgin abdomen. Hasson is preferred for patients with secondary abdomens, although for the particularly obese patient, this may be impractical. The Ethicon purple Hasson port may be used, keeping the purple outer sheath and exchanging the port itself for an extra long port. Alternatively, the extra-long port may be used alone (without the Hasson sheath); however, this port comes only with a bladed trocar that must be deactivated when introducing the port by Hasson technique. The fascial incision ought not to be wider than the trocar. Compensation is made at the skin level, and then it is closed with mattress sutures to prevent an air leak.

If Veress entry is used on a previously entered abdomen, it ought to be placed in a location remote from the prior surgical site. This is primarily to avoid bowel injury related to adhesions, although preservation of normal appearances is an important goal in the avoidance of untoward bleeding.

In fact, effort should be made throughout laparoscopic surgery to reflect planes of tissue when it will become immediately useful to isolate critical anatomy, and not before. Additionally, minimize instrument exchanges to keep the momentum and pace of dissection. The reason is that tissues, when left alone for a period of time, become stained with blood, which obscures the direction and leaves the surgeon with only memory, imagination, or the need to repeat exposure. This leads to aimless dissection, and mishap.

During trocar placement, particularly for pelvic surgery, pay attention to the anterior abdominal wall for the epigastric vessels. These are much easier to visualize during the extraperitoneoscopic method. Location of the femoral artery by the inguinal ligament is a good landmark for identifying the source and likely course of the inferior epigastric vessels during a transperitoneal laparoscopic approach. Occasionally, in thin patients, the vessels may be seen through the peritoneum. Transillumination of the abdominal wall with the laparoscope, in contrast, rarely identifies the inferior epigastrics. The preperitoneal approach to pelvic surgery deserves mention here: this technique is excellent for direct visualization of the inferior epigastric vessels. The operator is cautioned, however, to create the preperitoneal space with a balloon dilator (kidney-shaped; OMS-PDB2, US Surgical, Norwalk, CT) *slowly under laparoscopic vision* so that minor adjustments may be made to properly direct the balloon and prevent unnecessary nuisance hemorrhage.

Monopolar electrocautery may be used safely at distances from essential tissues to prophylactically coagulate tiny vessels throughout the course of dissection. The monopolar electrocautery cord may be connected to either the robotic hook instrument or the robotic "hot" scissors instrument.

Bipolar electrocautery may be used either prophylactically or to coagulate small bleeding vessels when the vessels are adjacent to essential tissues in need of preservation. The robotic Precise bipolar forceps and the robotic Maryland type bipolar forceps accommodate bipolar electrocautery, and they are excellent tools for this purpose.

As a matter of economy of motion, it often makes sense to maintain one working instrument arm with a grasping forceps that also has bipolar electrocautery capability and to maintain a second working instrument arm with either a hook or scissors connected to monopolar electrocautery. Such a setup allows for presentation of tissues with one arm, and cutting or dissection with the second arm, while affording minor hemostasis as needed.

The laparoscopic LigaSure Vessel Sealing System (Valleylab/Tyco, Boulder, CO) is a unique bipolar cautery with crush action within the jaws of the instrument. It comes in 5- and 10-mm sizes, and it may be used by the assistant adjunctively to ligate vessels within tissue that would certainly bleed if only simply divided. These instruments handle vessels up to 4 and 7 mm, respectively, with a thermal spread factor of up to 4 mm for the larger instrument *(1)*. The Harmonic Scalpel (Ethicon EndoSurgery, Cincinnati, OH), ACE (Ethicon EndoSurgery), and SonoSurg (Olympus, Tokyo, Japan) are also very useful, particularly for wading through vascularized fatty tissues (e.g., the lateral wings of the bladder at the prostatic-vesical junction).

4. MINOR VENOUS BLEEDING

Direct pressure and patience is often all that is necessary for minor venous bleeding. In kidney surgery, a suction cannula (without application of suction) often works well. Sometimes pressure with a flap of raised tissue works well. Introduction of a piece of Surgicel or Nu-Knit (oxidized cellulose) works well to maintain direct pressure with an instrument atraumatically and to facilitate trigger of the extrinsic coagulation cascade. Increasing insufflation pressure temporarily may not be necessary if the bleeding is very minor, but it may be helpful for the more generous ooze. Consider identifying a discrete small vessel that may be accessed and clipped but do not convert a small nuisance into something uncontrollable. If possible, avoid dissecting in that exact spot for a short time until other nearby structures are properly exposed. If the bleeding is in a critical area of dissection, accept the bleeding by using suction to clear the field, and expose what is necessary to ultimately include or exclude the bleeding site.

Do not clip blindly into the adrenal or pancreas! It is unlikely that the hemorrhage will stop with this maneuver, and in the latter case, fistulization or ductal injury is risked.

In prostate surgery, if there is minor oozing from the vascular pedicle or Denonvilliers fascia about the posterior bladder neck or seminal vesicles, direct pressure will never be adequate. Bipolar electrocautery is the primary solution to these nuisances. Increasing insufflation pressure temporarily may be very helpful if the primary hemostatic maneuvers are not immediately adequate.

5. MAJOR VENOUS BLEEDING

There is a tendency to drop exposure as soon as bleeding is noted. Don't! Place pressure directly on the bleeding vessel. If it seems useful, use a flap of tissue to help broaden the pressure there—a suction cannula is usually the best instrument for this. Next, raise the insufflation pressure to 20 mmHg. Then, think honestly and quickly about how to regain control. If it is apparent that safe repair is not possible robotically/laparoscopically, convert to open without hesitation. If safe repair looks feasible, consider the following.

Certain anatomic locations lend themselves better to different techniques. If it is the dorsal penile vein that is bleeding during radical prostatectomy, rather than use the suction cannula for direct pressure, place tension on the Foley catheter such that the balloon draws on the prostate. Temporary tourniquet on the penis also may be helpful. Next, expose the minimum necessary on the injured side and the contralateral side to place a suture ligature. Have the assistant use the suction cannula to manipulate the prostate from side to side and remove blood from field of view. A second or third stitch may be necessary under such circumstances, but the bleeding virtually always stops with this approach. Once the dorsal vein is controlled, move on to the prostatic–vesical junction and leave any remaining anterior apical dissection until after the pedicles are taken.

In the case of renal vein injury during radical nephrectomy, what gets done next depends in part upon how much of the renal hilum remains to be isolated. One option is to repair the vein with a figure-eight suture. Another is to rapidly complete the vein exposure necessary to place a stapler across it, including the bleeding point. Usually, the artery has not yet been exposed at this point, and the artery should be identified fairly quickly after such a maneuver to prevent congestion of the specimen and oozing from otherwise unimportant tributaries. Another alternative is to wade quickly superiorly and inferiorly to the vein (if not already done) until the psoas muscle is seen on either side. This may be done with pressure maintained on the renal vein. In so doing, it may be presumed that the artery is within the central wad of tissue, and a stapler may be fired across the wad, taking vein and artery together. Although this maneuver is not very pleasing from an aesthetic standpoint, and it is not advocated for elective dissection, it has been shown to be safe—no arteriovenous fistulas have been reported in the short term *(2)*.

In the case of renal vein injury during partial nephrectomy, repair of the vein becomes mandatory if salvage of the kidney remains a priority. (Note that accessory veins may be ligated with impunity provided that the main renal vein is intact because unlike arterial inflow, there is collateral venous outflow.) A figure-eight suture is the only reasonable solution. Hold pressure broadly with an instrument in the nondominant hand and raise insufflation pressure. Have a needle holder swapped into the dominant hand. Have a suture passed to the needle holder. Next, have the assistant use suction to clear the field of view, and use the cannula to help apply pressure on the vein while the operator gets organized with the suture. The simplest maneuver is to gently grab the vein at the venotomy site with a curved pickups (e.g., Maryland), thereby stopping the flow of blood and stabilizing the vein for suture placement. Consideration may be given to use of the laparoscopic Yasergil vascular clamps (Aesculap, Tuttlingen, Germany) to partially occlude the vein proximally and distally in a wedge manner about the venotomy. The assistant at the patient's bedside must be facile with the application and removal of these clips if this is elected. Then, under better control, a 4-0 or 5-0 Prolene stitch on a cardiovascular needle may be used to suture the venotomy closed. A fourth robotic arm, if available, may follow the suture and hold both ends upward on gentle tension. A surgeon's knot is advisable, but take care not to break the suture! *Pay attention to the response of the suture while it is being pulled and continually readjust the hold on the suture such that the needle holders are close to the knot point.* Alternatively, a long suture may be used with the intention of performing an extracorporeal knot tie; however, this is not recommended. The assistant must be perfectly facile with this technique, because there is no room for error; Prolene tends not to slip down easily with a knot pusher; and gentle constant tension must be maintained without tearing the vein.

6. MINOR ARTERIAL BLEEDING

The most commonly injured vessels are the inferior epigastrics. The robotic lens may not swing easily to this site, and it is often necessary to visualize and control this problem manually by disengaging the camera from the camera arm. Usually, this injury occurs during port placement (in which case the robot has not yet been docked). A temporizing figure-eight suture through skin and full thickness abdominal wall using 0-Prolene over a ray-tech bolster (on the exterior) usually suffices until time to closure. Alternatively, a fascial closure device may be used to place a permanent figure-eight stitch about the vessel (under the level of the skin). However tempting it is to use bipolar electrocautery to control this bleeding, this technique often fails, particularly if transperitoneal. If the vessel can be seen easily, consider controlling it with a clip.

Other intra-abdominal minor arteries may be grasped and clipped to control. Again, use only 10-mm, or medium/large, or large clips. Do not use 5-mm clips except in children—they do not purchase well, and release from the clip applier is often awkward and traumatic.

7. MAJOR ARTERIAL BLEEDING

If it is the renal artery during a nephrectomy, grasp the vessel, and clip to ligate. Do not grab the artery of a clipped vessel (including the artery on the specimen), because there is risk that the clips will fall off and bleeding may ensue. If there is a minor sharp nick in a major artery, primary suture repair by placement of a Prolene stitch may be considered. Apply direct pressure and place the stitch, or control the artery proximally and distally (using Yasergil vascular clamps if needed), and then place the stitch. If arterial clamping is necessary, consider heparinization and consultation with a vascular surgeon. If it is apparent that safe repair is not possible robotically/laparoscopically, convert to open without hesitation.

8. ELECTIVE HEMOSTASIS

8.1. Partial Nephrectomy

Case selection according to tumor location, tumor size, and skill levels of the surgeon, assistant, and nursing staff are paramount for a good outcome. Next, all of the necessary equipment must be in the room, opened and ready to use at a moment's notice.

For renal cortical tumors, exophytic in appearance and extending no deeper than 0.5 cm (the cortico-medullary line), hemostasis of the fossa may be handled with several different kinds of energy sources. The argon beam coagulator or the Harmonic Scalpel work well (3). Tumors extending deep to the cortico-medullary line are surrounded by vessels of significantly larger caliber, and the operator must be ready to exercise suture control. Although the superficial lesions may be attempted without gaining control of the renal hilum, the deeper tumors must not be touched without this control.

A preoperative computed tomography angiogram is helpful to determine the number of vessels supplying the kidney (4,5). Multiple different approaches have been applied to renal hilar control during laparoscopic partial nephrectomy, including clamping of the renal artery alone, clamping of renal artery and vein separately, and mass clamping of the central wad, including both renal artery and vein without their skeletonization. We are currently investigating the utility of endovascular hilar control to avoid dissection of the hilum altogether. Unlike open surgery, it is imperative that the working field be made perfectly bloodless to ensure that adequate margins of resection are well visualized and that needle placement is precise.

I skeletonize both artery and vein, double clamp the renal artery (Yasergil/Aesculap) and single clamp the vein. It is helpful to remove all perirenal fat and expose the entire kidney, thereby disrupting collateral blood supply before clamping of the renal hilum. The Harmonic Scalpel is particularly good for wading through this perirenal fat hemostatically. Often, the perirenal fat is caked onto the renal capsule (even in areas that are clearly not involved with tumor), and it is sometimes necessary to enter the renal capsule to displace the fat. This tends to make a bloody mess and adds to the complexity of exposure, incision, and reconstruction, although as long as the renal parenchyma is not fractured this in itself is not dangerous from standpoint of total blood loss.

Control of the tumor during resection is important and difficult. A handle may be made by placement of a figure-eight stitch either through the kidney just under the tumor or next to it (with an air knot) (6). This suture is placed just before renal hilar clamping, and in my experience it causes no significant bleeding. Others have fashioned a sling to stabilize the kidney during tumor resection (7). I resect the tumor by cutting sharply with curved scissors into the healthy renal parenchyma taking care to observe the parenchyma with each cut. Generally, tumors distant from the hilum are excised from medial to lateral with the tumor retracted away from the cut line as the cut progresses. This approach ensures visualization of the normal parenchymal bed during resection. The first cut is always the best cut, and revisions are very difficult to endure from a reconstructive standpoint. Thus, although use of the Harmonic Scalpel for this aspect of the procedure offers hemostatic advantage, it clouds perception of the proper cut line. Ultrasound is frequently used by those performing laparoscopic partial nephrectomy to delineate margins in advance of incising the renal capsule, although I have not found this more helpful than simply judging size according to what is obvious by direct laparoscopic visualization of the tumor and correlation with preoperative renal imaging. Although intraoperative duplex allows for identification of blood vessels in the vicinity of the tumor, it offers absolutely no protective benefit from a hemostatic standpoint. (I reserve intraoperative ultrasound for purposes of identifying the gross location of the renal lesion when exposure of the renal capsule is difficult and the tumor position is not immediately obvious).

To help keep the field bloodless, it is useful to raise the insufflation pressure to 20 mmHg for the duration of tumor resection and renal reconstruction. Once the kidney is reconstructed, the insufflation pressure is reduced to 5-7 mmHg to test the repair for hemostasis. Porcine models for examination of gas embolism during laparoscopic partial nephrectomy have shown no embolism at insufflation pressures as high as 30 mmHg unless argon beam coagulation was added (without a vent, at final pressures ranging 30–50 mmHg) *(8)*. This highlights the utility of renal vein clamping, not only to prevent back bleeding but also to serve as a prophylaxis against gas embolization. It also highlights the importance of venting the abdomen during use of the argon beam coagulator if this procedure is used as an adjunct.

About access: It is my view that hand-assisted techniques frustrate proper suturing reconstruction of the renal parenchyma, although others have clearly demonstrated its utility *(9)*. For those not quite fascicle with straight laparoscopic techniques, it may be useful to use a hand-assisted approach to isolate the anatomy before converting to robotic tumor resection and parenchymal reconstruction. The hand port (Ethicon EndoSurgery LapDisc) may be used to hold the 12-mm port for the robotic camera arm by dialing the diaphragm down to size. As for final impact upon total recovery, length of stay, or pain, it probably makes little difference whether the approach is purely laparoscopic (and robotic) or hand-assisted. However, *the angle of approach* to the tumor is critically important to a good outcome. Thus, a posterior tumor dictates a retroperitoneoscopic approach, and a superior-anterior lesion dictates a transperitoneal approach *(10)*.

Various suturing techniques have been described previously. I have found satisfactory use of Nu-Knit pledgets and Lapra-Ty clips (Ethicon EndoSurgery) on 0-Vicryl suture with a large tapered needle (CT or CT-X) for creating a tight pucker of the renal parenchyma. The pledget and clip are preloaded 2.5 in. from the tail end of the suture, cut to a total length of 7.5 in. The assistant must be practiced in stabilizing the kidney for suture needle placement, and placement of the Lapra-Ty or Hem-o-Lok (Weck/Teleflex Medical, Research Triangle Park, NC) clips. A robotic fourth arm may help stabilize the kidney during suture placement, but it does not replace the assistant entirely. It is important not to fracture the renal capsule as the kidney is pushed opposite the draw of the suture with the clip applier. Also, care must be made not to catch a piece of the pledget in these clips, because they then would not close properly. Other surgeons use a similar method, including a prerolled "cigar" of Surgicel in the fossa. The sutures are then tied over this bolster, which places downward pressure into the crater *(11)*. I find that the cigar method only costs valuable ischemic time without contributing much more to hemostasis than sutures and clips alone. If repair of the collecting system is necessary, simple running suture with 4-0 Vicryl on an RB-1 needle, tied without clips, works well.

Laparoscopic-assisted percutaneous radiofrequency coagulation of renal tumors has been performed just before tumor excision. This promising technique has facilitated tumor resection by minimizing blood loss, and it has preserved tumor architecture for accurate pathologic diagnosis *(12)*. Neither radiofrequency coagulation nor cryoablation have entered into mainstream renal tumor management as solitary treatment because of imperfect and unpredictable margins of treatment and a lack of long-term follow-up *(13)*. This is particularly true for larger (>3 cm) or endophytic tumors *(14)*. Similarly, neoadjuvant energy ablation has not become vogue.

Sealants should not be depended upon as a solitary means of obtaining hemostasis, although it apparently reduces chances of hemorrhage after reconstruction is complete *(15,16)*. Sealants have evolved to be considered an imperative adjunct; however, it should be recognized that there are no data on toxicity to renal parenchyma, nor is there a randomized controlled study demonstrating a clear benefit over suture hemostasis alone.

C. C. Abbou and colleagues have used "crepes" made of Surgicel filled with Colle Chirurgicale Cardial (gelatin, resorcinol, and formaldehyde; Bard, Saint-Etienne, France), then packed and soldered them in place with bipolar electrocautery. Remarkably large, deep renal defects may be handled adequately with this technique.

I have found success with BioGlue Surgical Adhesive (CryoLife, Inc., Kennesaw, GA). When the bovine serum albumin and glutaraldehyde mix, they form an impervious barrier almost instantly. The minimum anastomotic burst strength for this compound is 300 mmHg *(17)*. Its direct application to tissues may result in significant inflammation, edema, and toxic necrosis (which may be beneficial in establishing negative cancer margins), although there is a theoretical concern that these toxic effects may compromise integrity of the suture repair of these tissues *(18)*. In a clinical study of patients with type A thoracic aortic dissection randomized to surgical repair alone versus surgery with BioGlue as an adjunct, there was no statistically significant difference in mortality, although BioGlue patients required fewer pledgets, hemostatic agents, and makeup stitches compared with the control group *(19)*. One disadvantage is that the gun for this glue must be fired rapidly to push the

mixture down the relatively long laparoscopic applicator before it solid-
ifies within the applicator itself. If the flow is stopped at all, it clogs, and
a new applicator must be used. Final bond strength takes 2 min *(19)*.

FloSeal (Baxter Corporation, Mississauga, ON, Canada) is the
hemostatic agent now most in vogue in renal surgery. Collagen-deprived
granules (gelatin) and topical thrombin conforms to the wound. The
granules swell approximately 20% within 10 min of application, and
they restrict the flow of blood. Blood percolating through the spaces is
exposed to high concentration thrombin, which converts fibrinogen to
fibrin and forms clot around the mechanically stable granule matrix. It is
reabsorbed within 6 to 8 weeks *(20)*.

Tisseel VH (Baxter Corporation) is another hemostatic agent that
consists of fibrinogen, calcium, aprotinin, and thrombin. The components must be prepared with the warming kit supplied, and they must
be used within 4 h of its preparation. This awkward, in-operating room
preparation, has rendered the agent unpopular. QuikClot (Z-Medica,
Wallingford, CT), an adsorbent, is significantly easier to use and it is
under investigation (*(21)*; see Table 1).

8.2. Radical Prostatectomy

With modern-day techniques to control the dorsal venous complex,
this is usually not the source for most of the bleeding during radical open
surgery. Rather, it is the complex of finer veins that are disrupted that lead
to cumulative losses over time. For this reason, the pneumoperitoneum
established during laparoscopic and robotic prostatectomy is responsible
for the dramatic reduction in blood losses appreciable. Although an insufflation pressure of 15 mmHg is generally more than adequate, do not
hesitate to temporarily raise the pressure to 20 mmHg when there is
an annoying ooze to contend with. Even patients with moderate chronic
obstructive pulmonary disease or congestive heart failure can tolerate
transiently high insufflation pressures; venous return is generally not
impeded at pressures under 25 mmHg; and gas embolism is exceedingly
rare at such pressures. The economy of motion afforded by temporarily
raising the insufflation pressure, however, may make the difference
required to complete certain difficult anatomic dissections.

The robotic prostatectomist should quickly establish a comfortable
routine of wading through tissues, including relatively avascular and
vascular structures. The use of bipolar forceps on one instrument arm, and
monopolar hook cautery on another instrument arm is an excellent combination, particularly for wading through the space of Retzius, clearing the
superficial dorsal vein, clearing the fat away from the endopelvic gutters,
opening the endopelvic fascia, releasing the levator muscles, and coming

Table 1
Comparison of surgical adhesives

Adhesive	Manufacturer	FDA Approval	Mechanism	Comments
Bioglue Surgical Adhesive	CryoLife, Inc., Kennesaw, GA	Yes, for adjunctive use in repair of large vessels	Tissue fixative and barrier	Tissue toxicity unknown
Colle Chirur-gicale Cardial	Bard, Saint-Etienne, France	No	Tissue fixative and barrier	Tissue toxicity unknown
CoSeal	Baxter, Freemont, CA	Yes, for adjunctive use in vascular reconstruction	Mixture of polyethylene glycols seal tissue	Tissue toxicity unknown
FloSeal	Baxter Corporation, Mississauga, ON, Canada	Yes, as a hemostatic adjunct, but not for urologic use	Granules adsorb H_2O; thrombin converts fibrinogen to fibrin	Currently most in vogue; reabsorbs within 6 to 8 weeks
QuikClot	Z-Medica, Wallingford, CT	No	Synthetic volcanic-type granules adsorb H_2O; concentrates patient's own clotting factors	Exothermic reaction; chronic interstitial inflammation of renal tissue in contact
Tisseel VH	Baxter, Mississauga, ON, Canada	Yes, as a hemostatic adjunct in cardiopulmonary bypass, splenic injuries, and colostomy closure	Thrombotic agents applied	Requires warming preparation in operating room

through the bladder neck. Arguably, the back-and-forth use of these two instruments may be good for handling the vasa deferentia, seminal vesicles, and even the vascular pedicles. Alternatively, cold dissection may be performed using permanent or temporary clips via the manual 5-/12-mm assistant port, and scissors on the robotic instrument arm.

Handling the dorsal vein starts first with its exposure. Divide the puboprostatic ligaments and delineate the bulge of the vein complex riding anterior to the urethra. This helps establish a more accurate needle placement during suture ligation, and it allows for better purchase of the vein. Alternatively, either a mattress suture (under the vein and back through the puboprostatic ligaments), or a figure-8 stitch may help with purchase and ligation. The use of the LigaSure alone in this location is undependable for exacting hemostasis, and adjunctive suture ligation is often required. Finally, an endovascular stapler has been used by few for this structure with seemingly no major problem, although the potential for staple migration into the anastomotic site is theoretically bothersome.

Suture placement at the dorsal vein requires a certain calculated finesse. At least one needle holder should be used (I prefer two holders). Zero Vicryl on a CT-1 needle works very well. The simplest way to get started with this particular step is to place the needle flat on top of the prostate in simulation of its passage under the vein. Then, grasp the needle with the robotic needle holder close to the back end of the needle at exactly the angle created naturally by its lying on top of the prostate. (With experience, the needle angle becomes understood and it becomes unnecessary to actually place the needle on top of the prostate). For the right-handed surgeon passing a needle from right to left, move the prostate left with the left instrument to expose the right side of the groove between urethra and dorsal vein complex. Pass the needle into this groove exactly horizontal and push it straight across (i.e., do not use the wrist to turn the needle just yet). Then, release the exposure created by the left robotic instrument and have the assistant retract the left side of the prostate to the right with a suction cannula. A gentle turn of the right wrist should then reveal the needle tip emanating from the left groove where the left robotic instrument should be waiting to receive it. The suture should be rolled out from under the vein at this point. A double or triple surgeon's knot should be used. Alternatively, a square knot, converted to a hitch, then cinched down and reconverted to square may be used.

REFERENCES

1. Goldstein SL, Harold KL, Lentzner A et al (2002) Comparison of thermal spread after ureteral ligation with the Laparo-Sonic Ultrasonic Shears and the LigaSure System. J Laparoendosc Adv Surg Tech A 12:61–63.

2. Rapp DE, Orvieto MA, Gerber GS et al (2004) En bloc stapling of renal hilum during laparoscopic nephrectomy and nephroureterectomy. Urology 64:655–659.
3. Kaynan AM, McRae S, Winfield HN (2001) Laparoscopic enucleation of renal tumors. J Endourol 15 (Suppl 1): A134 (V7-P2).
4. Kaynan AM, Rozenblit AM, Figueroa KI et al (1999) Use of spiral computerized tomography in lieu of angiography for preoperative assessment of living renal donors. J Urol 161:1769–1775.
5. Rajamahanty SS, Simon R, Edye M et al (2005) Accuracy of three-dimensional CT angiography for preoperative vascular evaluation of laparoscopic renal donors. J Endourol 19:339–341.
6. Nguyen TT, Parkinson JP, Kuehn DM et al (2005) Technique for ensuring negative surgical margins during laparoscopic partial nephrectomy. J Endourol 19:410–415.
7. Chien GW, Orvieto MA, Chuang MS et al (2005) Use of suspension traction system for renal positioning during laparoscopic partial nephrectomy. J Endourol 19:406–409.
8. Weld KJ, Ames CD, Landman J et al (2005) Evaluation of intra-abdominal pressures and gas embolism during laparoscopic partial nephrectomy in a porcine model. J Urol 174:1457–1459.
9. Johnston WK, Montgomery JS, Seifman BD et al (2005) Fibrin glue V sutured bolster: lessons learned during 100 laparoscopic partial nephrectomies. J Urol 174:47–52.
10. Wright JL, Porter JR (2005) Laparoscopic partial nephrectomy: comparison of transperitoneal and retroperitoneal approaches. J Urol 174:841–845.
11. Ng CS, Gill IS, Ramani AP et al (2005) Transperitoneal versus retroperitoneal laparoscopic partial nephrectomy: patient selection and perioperative outcomes. J Urol 174:846–849.
12. Gettman MT, Bishoff JT, Su LM et al (2001) Hemostatic laparoscopic partial nephrectomy: initial experience with the radiofrequency coagulation-assisted technique. Urology 58:8–11.
13. Desai MM, Aron M, Gill IS (2005) Laparoscopic partial nephrectomy versus laparoscopic cryoablation for the small renal tumor. Urology 66(5 Suppl): 23–28.
14. Wagner AA, Solomon SB, Su LM (2005) Treatment of renal tumors with radiofrequency ablation. J Endourol 19:643–653.
15. Gill IS, Colombo JR, Frank I et al (2005) Laparoscopic partial nephrectomy for hilar tumors. J Urol 174:850–854.
16. Gill IS, Ramani AP, Spaliviero M et al (2005) Improved hemostasis during laparoscopic partial nephrectomy using gelatin matrix thrombin sealant. Urology 65: 463–466.
17. Gundry SR, Black K, Izutani H (2000) Sutureless coronary artery bypass with biologic glued anastomoses: preliminary in vivo and in vitro results. J Thorac Cardiovasc Surg 120:473–477.
18. Furst W, Banerjee A (2005) Release of glutaraldehyde from an albumin-glutaraldehyde tissue adhesive causes significant in vitro and in vivo toxicity. Ann Thorac Surg 79:1522–1528.
19. Summary of safety and effectiveness, CyroLife, Inc., BioGlue® Surgical Adhesive. http://www.fda.gov/cdrh/pdf/p010003b.pdf. Last accessed Nov. 8, 2005.
20. Summary of safety and effectiveness. http://www.fda.gov/cdrh/pdf/p990009b.pdf.
21. Margulis V, Matsumoto ED, Svatek R et al (2005) Application of novel hemostatic agent during laparoscopic partial nephrectomy. J Urol 174:761–764.

14 Complications of Robotic Surgery

Joseph R. Wagner and Caner Z. Dinlenc

1. INTRODUCTION

Over the past 25 years, technologic advances have dramatically improved urologic care in all subdivisions of urologic care. Extracorporeal shock wave lithotripsy, intracytoplasmic sperm injection, miniaturized endoscopy, surgical stapling devices, and laparoscopic nephrectomy/adrenalectomy are just a few examples. However, every new technologic advancement brings with it a new set of potential complications that must be considered, and robotic surgery is no exception.

Multiple studies have demonstrated that robotics can enable laparoscopically naïve surgeons to perform complex minimally invasive procedures with a shorter learning cure (1–3). Nonetheless, we firmly believe robotic surgery remains a remarkable laparoscopic tool, but the procedures themselves remain laparoscopic at heart. As long as robotic surgery entails trocar insertion and insufflation, the surgeon will continue to require an understanding of laparoscopic techniques, physiology, and complications. Many adverse outcomes can be prevented with thoughtful, preoperative planning, attention to detail during surgery, and proper postoperative care.

2. PATIENT SELECTION

Patient selection begins with a thorough history and physical examination. Comorbidities should be assessed preoperatively, with the physiologic changes unique to laparoscopic surgery kept in mind. For example, an obese patient with obstructive pulmonary disease and CO_2 retention may be difficult to ventilate with resultant hypercapnia during

From: *Current Clinical Urology: Urologic Robotic Surgery*
Edited by: J. A. Stock, M. P. Esposito, and V. J. Lanteri © Humana Press, Totowa, NJ

laparoscopy *(4)*. Before renal surgery, radiographic studies should be carefully examined for mass size and location, level of the renal hilum, renal vein or caval involvement, duplicated renal vessels, retro-aortic renal veins, on so on. These factors allow the surgeon to anticipate minor anatomic anomalies. Similarly, the presence of a median lobe during prostatectomy and the exact location of a ureteral tumor are critical pieces of information to have before a prostatectomy or distal ureterectomy.

The most favorable patients, especially during the initial learning phase, include those who are relatively thin and that have virgin abdominal cavities. Obese patients can be a significant challenge because excessive adipose tissue can make dissection tedious and difficult *(5,6)*. In addition, obesity increases the risk complications during laparoscopic surgery, particularly with the Trendelenberg/lithotomy position required for pelvic procedures *(7)*. Multiple prior abdominal surgeries predispose to intraperitoneal adhesions, which are time-consuming to lyse and increase the risk of visceral injury. Patients with extremely muscular abdominal walls have reduced abdominal wall compliance that reduces the working space and may limit exposure. As the surgeon's experience grows, patients with relative contraindications become more amenable to a robotic approach.

3. PREOPERATIVE PREPARATION

Patients should be appropriately informed of the surgeon's experience, the risks and benefits of robotic surgery versus standard laparoscopy verses open surgery, and other therapeutic options. In the event that the procedure is one of the first five for the surgeon, the use of proctor/mentor or similarly experienced colleague is highly recommended and may be required by the hospital's credentialing body. This circumstance should be discussed openly with the patient. Preoperative discussions should always include the caveat that conversion to an open procedure is possible. *Consent must include permission for open surgery.* Although robot malfunctions are rare, we also have a discussion with the patient as to whether it would be best to proceed with a laparoscopic or open approach in the face of an intraoperative malfunction, depending on the surgical case. Anticoagulants, including herbals, are discontinued preoperatively. A type and screen should be obtained. Although intraoperative bowel complications are rare, we still conservatively have all our patients perform a bowel preparation with clear liquids and magnesium citrate the day before surgery *(8)*. In addition, an empty bowel helps maximize working space and allows for more comfortable dissection. The patient should have nothing to eat or drink by mouth after midnight except for a sip of water with medications the morning of surgery.

4. SURGERY

Robotic surgical procedures have many of the same complications as their open-surgery counterparts (e.g., rectal injury during prostatectomy, inferior vena cava injury during nephrectomy), and it is beyond the scope of this chapter to address the myriad of potential surgical complications that can occur during specific procedures. Rather, we identify issues common to all robotic procedures that must be kept in mind during surgery to avoid complications.

Before induction of general anesthesia and endotracheal intubation, pneumatic antiembolic stockings are applied. After induction of anesthesia, a nasogastric/orogastric tube and a Foley catheter are used to keep the stomach and bladder decompressed. Prophylactic antibiotics are administered. For renal procedures, the patient is positioned in semilateral decubitus position at a 45° angle, by using gel pads to support the side of the pathology. A padded armrest is used to support the upper arm. An axillary roll is not required using the semilateral position. The lower leg is flexed, and the upper leg is extended with pillows placed in between. To allow the patient to be rolled intraoperatively from a near supine position to the full flank position, 3-in. cloth tape is wrapped over the patient and passed under the operating room table several times to secure the patient's head, shoulders, chest, hips, and legs. Upper and lower body warming blankets are used to maintain core body temperature throughout the case. The surgical field from nipples to pubis and laterally to the mid-axillary line should be shaved.

For pelvic procedures, the patient is placed in a modified lithotomy position. Heparin has been shown to be safe during radical prostatectomy, and because of the increased incidence of deep venous thrombosis with pelvic procedures, we administer 5,000 units of heparin subcutaneously in addition to placing pneumatic stockings (9). The buttock is placed at the end of the table to allow access to the rectum if necessary. The feet and lower legs are placed in padded stirrups, and the lower extremities are "dropped" so the hip is only slightly flexed. A small foam pad is placed around the patient's hands, and both upper extremities are well padded before they are tucked at the patient's sides. Velcro straps (or tape) can be placed in an X configuration across the chest, or shoulder bolsters can be placed, to support the patient in Trendelenberg. *Extreme care* should be taken during positioning to avoid neurologic injuries (femoral, obturator, peroneal, brachial) and pressure sores/contusions that can occur with inappropriate positioning (10). These concerns are more acute in the early phase of the surgeon's learning curve as the operative may approach be several hours longer than anticipated. The robot is then brought into the field between the patient's legs.

Although most anesthesiologists are comfortable with short laparoscopic procedures, such as cholecystectomy and hernia repair, they may be less versed in major, longer laparoscopic cases and inappropriately treat the patient as they would an open case. Given the decreased blood loss, decreased insensible loss, and decreased urine output due to insufflation pressures, this can result in fluid overload. Avoid nitrous inhalants because they can cause bowel distension, resulting in decreased exposure. Insufficient ventilation can result in hypercapnia with pulmonary arrest or fatal arrythmias. A multi-institutional review by Gill et al. (11) revealed that 35% of complications were due to the physiologic changes that occur during laparoscopy. *Open communication* before and during the surgery with the anesthesia team will avoid many of these complications.

Initial access and trocar placement during laparoscopic surgery can be the cause of significant morbidity. The choice of Veress needle or Hasson access for initial access should be made by surgeon experience, preference, and patient factors. A Hasson technique should certainly be used in patients with a history of prior abdominal surgery (12). When placing robotic and assistant trocars, transilluminate the abdomen to avoid major vessels, particularly the epigastric (13). Be sure the incision is long enough to permit the trocar without undue pressure on the skin, and trocars should be placed at a slight angle toward the surgical site. Excessive subcutaneous dissection should be avoided because this enables subcutaneous CO_2 infiltration. Proper trocar placement, neither too near nor too far apart, is critical in robotic surgery. Placing the trocars too far apart may inhibit the surgeon's ability to reach the surgical site; placing them too close may cause the robot arms to clash. In obese patients, consider moving the trocars closer to the surgical site to compensate for the loss of length due to the thick abdominal wall. Port placement for widefield dissections such as bilateral pelvic lymph nodes can be frustrating. The robot's primary design was to aid in microsurgical reconstruction (i.e., coronary vessels), not sweeping abdominal maneuvers. The lateral extreme ranges of motion required for bilateral pelvic node dissection require a more cephalad placement of ports, which may make reaching the 6 o'clock urethra difficult or impossible.

Rectal injuries can be categorized into perforating trauma or thermal injury, resulting in delayed sloughing. The former injury is easy to envision, especially considering lack of tactile sensation during robotic cases. Interestingly, there has been no data to suggest that this actually happens with regularity. When suspected, a well lubricated rectal Bouge can be introduced to closely inspect and grade the injury. Small lesions can be closed primarily if there is limited spillage or the bowel is prepared. Larger injuries should be handled with proximal diversion after closure. Thermal injuries inevitably result from the use of cautery, either monopolar or bipolar. These may be difficult to appreciate, and they can present as a colovesical fistula in the early postoperative period. Thus, the only way to avoid these injuries is to avoid use any cautery near intestinal serosa. Generally, small bleeders tamponade with time, and larger bleeders can be ligated with an absorbable figure-eight suture.

Be sure none of the robot arms are in contact with the patient. This should be assessed periodically, particularly when the robot is at the extremes of its range. For example, trying to look at the anterior abdominal wall with a 30° down lens might place the camera against the patient's face or endotracheal tube. Surgeon, assistant, and anesthesiologist should all be vigilant of the robot's position. Because of the relative lack of "touch" and the concentration on the surgical site, the surgeon is often unaware that one of his or her arms/instruments in against pelvic bone or a vital structure. Careful attention by the assistant and open communication can avoid annoying minor bleeding from the pubis or a major iatrogenic injury to an adjacent organ.

Bleeding is not an uncommon complication of laparoscopic procedures *(14)*. These injuries can occur due to thermal injury, blunt trauma, or stapler/clip misadventure. Depending on the situation, pressure, endoscopic clips or staplers, fibrin sealants, Surgicel, temporarily raising the insufflation pressure, or free suturing techniques can generally salvage the situation. However, one should not hesitate to obtain adequate assistance when necessary or to convert to an open procedure.

Once the procedure is completed, the pneumoperitoneum should be decreased to assess for adequate hemostasis. *All trocars should be removed under laparoscopic visualization to assess for bleeding.* Significant bleeding can be controlled with fulguration or endoscopic suturing with a Carter-Thomason needle *(15)*. Care should be taken to completely close all indicated port sites (≥ 10 mm for a cutting trocar) to prevent herniation *(16)*.

Finally, the patient should be examined for signs of significant subcutaneous emphysema, which can be associated with pneumomediastinum or pneumothorax. The presence of diffuse crepitus is associated with mucosal absorption and resultant laryngeal obstruction in a patient in whom hyperventilation may be required to expel excess CO_2. Therefore, extubation in this setting must be controlled: lack of cuff leak around endotracheal tube with a deflated balloon, chest X-ray evidence of pneumomediastinum, direct visualization of laryngeal collapse, or baseline pulmonary insufficiency are all indications for delayed extubation. Lengthy procedures, increased number of trocars, multiple trocar insertion attempts, and high insufflation pressures are all risk factors for CO_2 absorption *(17,18)*.

Needless to say, initial robotic cases can be lengthy, and long operative times increase the chance of positioning issues, pulmonary complications, rhabdomyolysis, and so on. Observing an experienced surgeon for multiple procedures, carefully choreographing and practicing the procedure inanimately with your team, and obtaining a proctor during your initial experience decrease surgical morbidity considerably.

5. CONCLUSIONS

In any surgery, diligent preoperative assessment and preparation, thoughtful operative planning and attention to detail during surgery, and open communication with the operative team will avoid most perioperative complications. The majority of complications during robotic surgery can be addressed laparoscopically, particularly with increased surgeon experience and skills. However, one should not hesitate to enlist the aid of a more experienced robotic/laparoscopic surgeon or convert to open surgery when the situation warrants.

REFERENCES

1. Ahlering TE, Skarecky D, Lee D et al (2003) Successful transfer of open surgical skills to a laparoscopic environment using a robotic interface: initial experience with laparoscopic radical prostatectomy. J Urol 170:1738.
2. Perer E, Lee DI, Ahlering T et al (2003) Robotic revelation: laparoscopic radical prostatectomy by a nonlaparoscopic surgeon. J Am Coll Surg 197:693.
3. Yohannes P, Rotariu P, Pinto P et al (2002) Comparison of robotic versus laparoscopic skills: is there a difference in the learning curve? Urology 60:39.
4. Sprung J, Whalley DG, Falcone T et al (2002) The impact of morbid obesity, pneumoperitoneum, and posture on respiratory system mechanics and oxygenation during laparoscopy. Anesth Analg 94:1345.
5. Lamvu G, Zolnoun D, Boggess J et al (2004) Obesity: physiologic changes and challenges during laparoscopy. Am J Obstet Gynecol 191:669.
6. Mendoza D, Newman RC, Albala D et al (1996) Laparoscopic complications in markedly obese urologic patients (a multi-institutional review). Urology 48:562.
7. Stone J, Dyke L, Fritz P et al (1998) Hemodynamic and hormonal changes during pneumoperitoneum and Trendelenburg positioning for operative gynecologic laparoscopy surgery. Prim Care Update Ob Gyns 5:155.
8. Bishoff JT, Allaf ME, Kirkels W. et al (1999) Laparoscopic bowel injury: incidence and clinical presentation. J Urol 161:887.
9. Sieber PR, Rommel FM, Agusta VE et al (1997) Is heparin contraindicated in pelvic lymphadenectomy and radical prostatectomy? J Urol 158:869.

10. Wolf JS Jr, Marcovich R, Gill IS et al (2000) Survey of neuromuscular injuries to the patient and surgeon during urologic laparoscopic surgery. Urology 55:831.

11. Gill IS, Kavoussi LR, Clayman RV et al (1995) Complications of laparoscopic nephrectomy in 185 patients: a multi-institutional review. J Urol 154:479.

12. Lecuru F, Leonard F, Philippe JJ et al (2001) Laparoscopy in patients with prior surgery: results of the blind approach. JSLS 5:13.

13. Hurd WW, Amesse LS, Gruber JS et al (2003) Visualization of the epigastric vessels and bladder before laparoscopic trocar placement. Fertil Steril, 80:209.

14. Parsons JK, Varkarakis I, Rha KH et al (2004) Complications of abdominal urologic laparoscopy: longitudinal five-year analysis. Urology 63:27.

15. Ortega II (1996) The Carter-Thomason needle suture passer to correct cannula-induced defects and vascular injuries in the abdominal wall during laparoscopy. J Am Assoc Gynecol Laparosc 3:S37.

16. Holzinger F and Klaiber C (2002) Trocar site hernias. A rare but potentially dangerous complication of laparoscopic surgery]. Chirurg 73:899.

17. Siu W, Seifman BD, Wolf JS Jr (2003) Subcutaneous emphysema, pneumome-diastinum and bilateral pneumothoraces after laparoscopic pyeloplasty. J Urol 170:1936.

18. Murdock CM, Wolff AJ, Van Geem T (2000) Risk factors for hypercarbia, subcu-taneous emphysema, pneumothorax, and pneumomediastinum during laparoscopy. Obstet Gynecol 95:704.

15 Policy Guidelines for Robot-Assisted Surgery in Urology

Ralph Madeb, Joy Knopf, Gregory Oleyourryk, Louis Eichel, and John R. Valvo

1. INTRODUCTION

One of the qualities innate to almost all physicians is a yearning for betterment. To improve medical standards and the delivery of healthcare to their patients, clinical physicians strive daily for improvement. One of the stressors accompanying this goal, and one particular to surgeons, is the never-ending need to incorporate new technology into the surgical armamentarium. With the emergence of minimally invasive laparo-scopic, robotic, and endo-operative techniques, this technology has been the focus of many surgeons, in all specialties, worldwide. Borne with these advancements and their advantages are the challenges, ethical and otherwise, of incorporating surgical technology into our care of the sick. Currently, in the United States, each individual hospital is required to develop criteria and policies for granting clinical privileges to surgeons operating in the hospital. This requirement is usually deferred to either the medical director or the chief of the particular surgical service who verifies whether a respective surgeon is "credentialed" for that procedure. In turn, the hospital's medical staff office is required by the Joint Commission of Accreditation of Healthcare Organizations to verify the credentials and training of its practitioners to delineate clinical privileges. One of the primary reasons that this system came into existence was for credentialing the aging surgeons. It is well known that as we age, fine motor skills wane. Therefore, it was recommended that "as age advances, a

From: *Current Clinical Urology: Urologic Robotic Surgery*
Edited by: J. A. Stock, M. P. Esposito, and V. J. Lanteri © Humana Press, Totowa, NJ

physician should, from time to time scrutinize impartially, the state of his faculties; that he may determine, *bona fide*, the precise degree in which he is qualified to execute the active and multifarious offices of his profession." The process that materialized and that is described above is now standard practice across the nation. Unfortunately, this system was clearly not designed to address the introduction of new and revolutionary surgical techniques and machinery. What remains is the question, How do we credential surgeons with new surgical technology, in particular, robot-assisted surgery?

2. ROBOT-ASSISTED SURGERY

Robot-assisted surgery is the application of advanced computerized technology in the planning, performance, and follow-up of invasive surgical procedures. The Food and Drug Administration (FDA) approved the da Vinci Surgical System (Intuitive Surgical, Sunnyvale, CA) in April 2004 for use in several surgical areas, which included cardiac, urologic, and gynecologic surgery. The da Vinci Surgical System consists of a three-dimensional laparoscopic vision system and two or three robotic arms that can perform high-precision articulating movements with a variety of instruments. Both the vision system and the robotic arms are controlled by the surgeon in a "master/slave" relationship via a remote surgeon's console that houses the vision system and the telemanipulators for the robotic arms. The technology allows for more precise and anatomical dissection with outcomes equal to or better than conventional techniques in both academic and private practice-based settings *(1–5)* and in both laparoscopic- and nonlaparoscopic-trained surgeons *(6,7)*.

Robot-assisted surgery is not a mere extension of a surgeon's ability to perform open or laparoscopic surgery. The appropriate and safe use of this technology requires specialized training and experience. Although the FDA reviews the results of laboratory, animal, and human clinical testing, it does not develop or test products. Moreover, the FDA does not regulate who buys or uses the product or whether a physician is qualified to use the equipment. The ability to perform a surgical procedure is regulated by hospital-based credentialing policy. Credentialing is the systematic approach to the collection, review, and verification of a practitioner's professional qualification.

3. CREDENTIALING

Robot-assisted surgery may not be learned safely during a weekend course. Dedication, commitment, and unique cognitive and technical skills are required to transfer ability from an open or laparoscopic to a robotic setting. Currently, there are no widely accepted guidelines that define appropriate credentialing for robot-assisted urologic surgery.

The urologists at Rochester General Hospital have experience with >1,000 robot-assisted radical prostatectomies. This experience includes both performance of the operation and frequent proctoring of other surgeons' training in robot-assisted surgery. To the best of our knowledge, most institutions have embarked on robot-assisted surgical programs without the benefit of procedural guidelines for obtaining surgical privileges or credentialing a physician for robot-assisted surgery. Credentialing is considered on a case-by-case basis. Therefore, we tried to determine policy for credentialing and maintenance of credentials for robotic-assisted radical prostatectomy. The guidelines defined here propose criteria and processes for obtaining privileges for performing robot-assisted radical prostatectomy by using the da Vinci Surgical System. The use of this technology should be limited to the level of intervention already granted under the same privileges for advanced laparoscopic procedures. Special circumstances may arise where robot-assisted surgery may be appropriate for nonlaparoscopic open surgical procedures. Overall, we recommend a minimum of four cases be proctored before performing robotic surgery without guidance. Based on consensus opinion, four cases is a practical number and takes into account a surgeon's past operative experience, availability of appropriate proctors, and cost needed to embark upon a robotic program. More importantly, each proctor and trainee must determine whether additional cases may be required before performing these procedures independently.

We think that every institution that invests in the da Vinci Surgical System should consider establishing a robot-assisted surgical subcommittee of their existing credentialing committee. As with any surgical procedure, credentialing should be dictated by the policies of the local hospital or institution. To the best of our knowledge, and likely due to the newness of the technology, most institutions have embarked on robot-assisted surgical programs without the benefit of procedural guidelines for obtaining surgical privileges and credentialing for robot-assisted surgery. The purposed guidelines can serve as a template to such committees in an effort to provide direction for the successful launch of a new program or facilitation of success for an ongoing program.

3.1. Requirements

3.1.1. PHYSICIAN CREDENTIALING

1. The individual possesses full attending privileges to perform open radical prostatectomy before requesting privileges to perform robotic prostatectomy.

2. The physician must show evidence of attendance and successful completion of a hands-on training program in the use of the da Vinci surgical platform. The program must be at least *8 h* in duration. The physician must have at least 3 h of personal experience on the system during this course.

3. Evidence of a practical experience via an accredited fellowship or residency program and clinical experience in a minimum of *30* computer-assisted procedures using the da Vinci surgical platform may be substituted for steps 1 and 2.

4. The physician must show evidence of having observed at least *four clinical cases* using the robotic system.

5. The surgeon must be proctored until the surgeon demonstrates successful use of the robotic system and a minimum of *four cases must be proctored.*

6. In the absence of a credentialed proctor, a second surgeon who has met steps 1–4, may serve as a co-surgeon or as the proctor.

7. It is the responsibility of the applicant to obtain a suitable proctor. The proctor should have temporary *or* courtesy privileges to enhance the learning experience and must be appropriately credentialed to serve as a proctor by the Computer-Assisted Surgical Committee and the Chief of Service *before* serving as a proctor.

8. Requests for privileges will be reviewed by the Computer-Assisted Surgical Committee and Chief of Service, as per the By-Laws of the Medical and Dental Staff.

9. Other special circumstances may be considered on a case-by-case basis, subject to the review and recommendation of the Computer-Assisted Surgical Committee.

10. To obtain credentialing, a surgeon must anticipate 20 robotic cases per year.

11. To maintain credentialing, a surgeon must perform 20 robotic cases per year.

12. An interruption of computer-assisted surgery greater than or equal to 6 mo requires the review of credentialing by Computer-Assisted Surgical Committee at his or her institution.

3.1.2. Surgical Assistants (Nonphysician)

1. The physician to be assisted must have clinical privileges to use the da Vinci Surgical System.

2. Nonphysician staff must be designated Registered Nurse First Assistant, Nurse Practitioner, or Physician Assistant with hospital privileges.

3. The surgical assistant must have attended a hands-on training practicum (which can occur on-site at the local hospital) of at least *6 h.*

4. The surgical assistant *only* applies to the bedside assistant. The assistant *may not* operate the surgical console.

3.1.3. SURGICAL ASSISTANTS (ATTENDING PHYSICIANS)

1. The physician must be board-certified, board-eligible within his or her surgical specialty, or a resident/fellow in training.
2. The physician must have hospital privileges and meet criteria as specified in the By-Laws of the Department of Surgery and the Medical and Dental Staff.
3. The surgical assistant must have attended a hands-on training practicum (which can occur on-site at the local hospital) of at least *6 h*.
4. The surgical assistant *only* applies to the bedside assistant function.

3.1.4. MONITORING.

1. Ongoing clinical monitoring of cases performed using the da Vinci surgical platform should be conducted.
2. Surgical outcomes should be analyzed periodically.

3.1.5. RECOMMENDED

1. It is highly recommended that surgeons be trained as teams of two individuals.
2. Physicians in each trained team should be able to function as either the surgeon, or assistant.
3. The trained pairs can each be used to proctor their counterpart on the team for the purpose of complying with the foregoing policy and procedure.
4. Given the complexity of the technology and the procedures to be performed, it is preferable to have a specially trained and designated team of operating room personnel (robotic team) who scrub and circulate on robotic cases. This model is consistent with the pump team for cardiac surgical procedures.

4. CONCLUSIONS

In the era of evidence-based medicine, surgical competence is increasingly being defined by the volume of procedures needed for acceptable outcomes. This relationship has been demonstrated in the urologic literature with open radical prostatectomy where it has been shown that rates of postoperative and late urinary complications are significantly reduced if the procedure is performed in a high-volume hospital and by a surgeon who performs a high number of such procedures *(8,9)*. Studies in other disciplines have demonstrated that a caseload threshold exists beyond which adverse surgical outcomes decline for hospitals or surgeons. As a result of such studies, other disciplines already require a minimum number of procedures to obtain surgical privileges, maintain surgical privileges, or both *(10–13)*. The Society for Bariactric Surgery requires a 150-case minimum per year per institution and a 50-case minimum per year per surgeon to be recognized as a center of excellence *(14,15)*. The American Society for Gastrointestinal Endoscopy guidelines recommend a minimum number for each endoscopic procedure performed before competence can be assessed *(16)*. Although many think that quality is inherent in quantity, the frequency of a procedure is more that just a marker of quality. Experience gained through repetition may be an underrated aspect of a surgeon's technical ability. We recommended that a minimum number of robot-assisted cases be performed annually. Although the benefits of quantity of surgical procedures are controversial, idle motor skills wane faster than memories. Therefore, there is a growing demand for demonstrating of maintenance of competency by practicing surgeons.

The above-mentioned proposal was conceived with robotic-assisted radical prostatectomy in mind. It is important to note that many urologists have already used the da Vinci Surgical System in other pathologies of the urinary system, including kidney, bladder, and ureteral surgery. "Pay-for-performance" will soon require that urologists track outcomes. Because we introduced this topic, we must remember that the concept of high-quality surgical care is everyone's goal. Periodic review is mandatory to expose deficiencies and improve quality outcomes. Procedural credentialing is a privilege—not a right, and it serves to protect patients from practitioners whose skills are less than an acceptable standard. We propose these guidelines to assist urologists and their medical institutions with commencing a successful and safe transition from open to robot-assisted surgery.

Disclaimer: We propose these guidelines as an educational, professional medical group, and we are not intended to be, nor should we be viewed, as a credentialing body. The above-mentioned guidelines were based on our urologists' personal experiences, and are they not intended to serve as "standard of care" for any robot-assisted procedures. Although we view these guidelines as important to successful surgical outcomes, we do not warrant, guarantee, or otherwise promise that institutions who implement these guidelines will achieve positive surgical outcomes for any robot-assisted procedure.

REFERENCES

1. Ahlering TE, Eichel L, Edwards RA, Lee DI, Skarecky DW (2004) Robotic radical prostatectomy: a technique to reduce pT2 positive margins. Urology 64:1224.
2. Ahlering TE, Woo D, Eichel L, Lee DI, Edwards R, Skarecky DW (2004) Robot-assisted versus open radical prostatectomy: a comparison of one surgeon's outcomes. Urology 63:819.
3. Menon M, Tewari A, Peabody J (2003) Vattikuti Institute prostatectomy: technique. J Urol 169:2289.

4. Menon M, Hemal AK (2004) Vattikuti Institute prostatectomy: a technique of robotic radical prostatectomy: experience in more than 1000 cases. J Endourol 18:611.

5. Tewari A, Menon M (2003) Vattikuti Institute prostatectomy: surgical technique and current results. Curr Urol Rep 4:119.

6. Ahlering TE, Skarecky D, Lee D, Clayman RV (2003) Successful transfer of open surgical skills to a laparoscopic environment using a robotic interface: initial experience with laparoscopic radical prostatectomy. J Urol 170:1738.

7. Madeb R, Golijanin D, Knopf J et al (2007) Transition from open to robotic-assisted radical prostatectomy is associated with a reduction of positive surgical margins amongst private-practice-based urologists. J Robot Surg 1(2):145–149.

8. Begg CB, Riedel ER, Bach PB et al (2002) Variations in morbidity after radical prostatectomy. N Engl J Med 346:1138.

9. Bianco FJ, Riedel ER, Begg CB, et al (2005) Variations among high volume surgeons in rate of complications after radical prostatectomy: further evidence that technique matters. J Urol 173: 2099.

10. Chowdhury MM, Dagash H, Pierro A (2007) A systematic review of the impact of volume of surgery and specialization on patient outcome. Br J Surg, 94:145.

11. Chun FK, Briganti A, Antebi E, Graefen M, Currlin E, Steuber T et al (2006) Surgical volume is related to the rate of positive surgical margins at radical prostatectomy in European patients. BJU Int 98:1204.

12. Elting LS, Pettaway C, Bekele BN et al (2005) Correlation between annual volume of cystectomy, professional staffing and outcomes: a statewide, population-based study. Cancer 104:975.

13. Gammie JS, O'Brien SM, Griffith BP, Ferguson TB, Peterson ED (2007) Influence of hospital procedural volume on care process and mortality for patients undergoing elective surgery for mitral regurgitation. Circulation 115:881.

14. ASBS Bariatric Training Committee (2006) American Society for Bariatric Surgery's guidelines for granting privileges in bariatric surgery. Surg Obes Relat Dis 2:65.

15. American Society for Metabolic and Bariatric Surgery (2007) http://www.asbs.org/. Cited 23 Nov. 2007.

16. Sharma VK, Coppola AG Jr, Raufman JP (2005) A survey of credentialing practices of gastrointestinal endoscopy centers in the United States. J Clin Gastroenterol 39:501.

16 Anesthetic Considerations for Laparoscopic Procedures in Urology

Leslie M. Leaf, Daniel C. Leaf,
Robert S. Dorian, and Mark Hausdorff

1. INTRODUCTION

1.1. History of Laparoscopy

Laparoscopic techniques in surgery have garnered wide acceptance since their inception in the 1970s. An endoscopic approach has lead to a decrease in postoperative pain, shortened hospitalizations, decreased wound complications such as infection and dehiscence, improved cosmetic result, and a potential lower cost to the hospital per patient *(1)*. For these reasons, minimally invasive procedures are now a mainstream approach to many surgical diseases.

1.2. Indications in Urology

A wide range of laparoscopic procedures are being performed in urology: the evaluation and repair of an undescended testis, varicocelectomy, bladder suspension, pelvic lymphadenectomy, nephrectomy, partial nephrectomy including donor nephrectomy for transplant, nephrourereterectomy, adrenalectomy, prostatectomy, and cystectomy *(2)*. The endoscopic approach has direct perioperative and postoperative implications for the anesthesiologist and surgeon.

1.3. Issues in Urology

Procedures in urology differ from general laparoscopic techniques that address intra-abdominal pathology. Urologic procedures are unique

From: *Current Clinical Urology: Urologic Robotic Surgery*
Edited by: J. A. Stock, M. P. Esposito, and V. J. Lanteri © Humana Press, Totowa, NJ

because the organs in the genitourinary system are located in the extraperitoneal space. This necessitates extraperitoneal insufflation with a compressed gas such as carbon dioxide (CO_2) to gain access to the surgical site. The absorption of CO_2 into the systemic circulation is greatly increased from the extraperitoneal space, the implications of which are discussed later in this chapter.

Minimally invasive procedures have an impact on homeostasis. With many physiological changes that take place. Three specific issues the anesthesiologist must appreciate are; the pneumoperitoneum, the changes in the partial pressure of carbon dioxide ($PaCO_2$), and patient positioning a (3). The organ systems most affected are the cardiovascular, pulmonary, and endocrine. In order to maximize perioperative management, it is imperative to understand the hemodynamic and pulmonary changes that occur during laparoscopic surgery. Finally, the introduction of robotics in laproscopic surgery requires additional considerations for the anesthesiologist.

2. PHYSIOLOGICAL EFFECTS OF LAPAROSCOPIC SURGERY

2.1. Pneumoperitoneum

A pneumoperitoneum is created when a compressed gas such as CO_2 fills the abdomen. As a result, gas entering the space causes separation of the anterior abdominal wall off the organs below. This allows for the visualization of anatomical structures and adequate space to perform surgery. The pressure created due to the volume of gas trapped in a closed space exerts force on all structures. The most pertinent structures effected are the diaphragm, lungs, and major abdominal vessels, but there also are effects on the systemic circulation and endocrine system.

Significant alterations in hemodynamics occur as a result of peritoneal and extraperitoneal insufflation. Intra-abdominal pressure (IAP) greater than 10 mmHg is associated with a decrease in cardiac output (CO) (4). Most studies indicate a fall in CO between 10 and 30% during insufflation, regardless of the patient position (5,6). However, in healthy patients, American Society of Anesthesiology (ASA) class I and II, this fluctuation is well tolerated according to a study using venous oxygen saturation and lactate concentrations as a measure of tissue perfusion (7). In addition, an increase in systemic vascular resistance (SVR) may occur as well as an increase in arterial pressure (8,9). Hemodynamic changes are most pronounced during the initial phase of insufflation and typically are transient. The accepted mechanisms for the decrease in CO is a decrease in venous return due to pooling of blood in the distal extremities, caval compression and an increase in venous resistance (10,11).

Support for this mechanism has been established by a reduction in left ventricular end diastolic volume measured by transesophageal echocardiography *(12)*. Hemodynamic changes can be minimized by increasing circulating volume before the case or by placing the patient in the Trendelenburg position during the initial insufflation, both of which can increase venous return *(13–15)*.

An increase in SVR and arterial blood pressure has been attributed to catecholamines, the renin-angiotensin system, and vasopressin *(6,16–18)*. In addition to a neurohumoral response, a direct stimulation of peritoneal receptors leads to an additional release of vasopressin. In high-risk cardiac patients, hemodynamic changes may lead to serious sequela. The increase in afterload adds strain on an already dysfunctional myocardium. The calcium channel blocker nicardipine acts selectively on arterial resistance to lower SVR, and does not result in a decrease in venous return and may be helpful in certain situations *(19)*.

Dysrhythmias are another potential consequence of the pneumoperitoneum. The increase in intra-abdominal pressure may lead to vagal stimulation *(20)*. Sinus bradycardia is the most common response to increased vagal tone, and although rare, a nodal rhythm or asystole may occur. The recommended treatments for a bradycardic dysrhythmia are immediately decreasing or discontinuing insufflation for a brief period; increasing the depth of anesthesia; and if necessary, administering an anticholinergic, e.g. atropine or glycopyrrolate. Pretreatment with a vagolytic is not recommended.

2.2. CO_2 Absorption and Accumulation

The most commonly used gas in laparoscopy is CO_2. The absorption and accumulation of CO_2 are related to its diffusion and solubility properties. Diffusion occurs when a gas molecule passes through a membrane from a higher partial pressure to a lower partial pressure. When gas molecules arrive at a liquid gas interface, the properties of solubility dictate the movement of that gas. This is known as the diffusion capacity, which for CO_2 is 20.5 times that of oxygen *(21)*. During initial insufflation, the brain, liver, heart, and kidneys (vessel-rich tissues) preferentially receive the CO_2. As the buffering capacity of the blood becomes overwhelmed, the vessel poor tissues, e.g., muscle and subcutaneous tissue, act as reservoirs for this gas, which leads to a delayed increase in $PaCO_2$, often seen in longer laparoscopic surgeries. The deleterious effects of an unrecognized rise in $PaCO_2$ are respiratory acidosis, a decreased arrhythmia threshold, and cerebral vasodilatation.

Current studies suggest that there is an initial rise in $PaCO_2$ during laparoscopic procedures. This typically occurs within the first 15 to

30 min from the creation of the pneumoperitoneum *(3,22,23)*. Multiple mechanisms lead to an increase in $PaCO_2$. CO_2 absorption is a function of the surface area exposed to gas and blood flow to that region. Moreover, there is up to a 76% increase in absorption that occurs with extraperitoneal insufflation *(24)*. Absorption of gas may be the major factor leading to the rise in $PaCO_2$ in patients undergoing laparoscopy. Additionally, a decrease in pulmonary ventilation from the increased IAP occurs. This results in a decrease in functional residual capacity (FRC), which promotes the accumulation of CO_2. Monitoring patients' oxygen saturation and analyzing the capnograph are essential, whereas obtaining arterial blood gases may be helpful in certain situations. Studies have shown that in healthy spontaneously breathing patients, ASA class 1 and 2, there will be an increase in minute ventilation (Ve = RR × TV) by 3^L/min for each 1 mmHg increase in $PaCO_2$ to compensate for the hypercarbia. However, patients undergoing general anesthesia have an increased work of breathing due to the addition of dead space, drug induced ventilatory depression and a decrease in thoracopulmonary compliance, all of which may lead to an uncompensated accumulation in $PaCO_2$. Careful monitoring by the anesthesiologist is required and maintaining normocarbia via ventilator changes may be indicated.

The inert gases argon and helium have been evaluated for use in laparoscopic procedures as an alternative to CO_2. Regardless of the type of gas used, an increase in intra-abdominal pressure causes similar hemodynamic effects. The low blood gas solubility of argon and helium increases the potential for a gas embolism *(24,25)*. Nitrous oxide (N_2O) is another gas that may be used to create a pneumoperitoneum. Both N_2O and CO_2 may lead to hollow viscera distension because of their high diffusion capacities. However, N_2O tends to remain in the distended viscera for a longer period. In addition, its flammability, associated nausea and vomiting, postoperative abdominal pain, and reported ileus are all further disadvantages of N_2O. There are many advantageous reasons for using CO_2. It is nonflammable, readily diffuses across a membrane, and is efficiently buffered by the blood and removed by the lungs. Most importantly, the anesthesiologist has means to readily detect levels of $EtCO_2$ and $PaCO_2$.

2.3. Patient Positioning

Laparoscopic urologic surgeries are commonly performed in one of four positions: supine head down, supine head up, lateral decubitus, and lithotomy. The physiological changes that occur in these positions primarily affect the respiratory, cardiovascular, and nervous systems.

The respiratory system is affected in the head down position by a significant decrease in FRC and lung compliance. Those who are the most vulnerable to these pulmonary insults are neonates, the elderly, COPD and obese patients. The potential for hypoxemia in this position requires the anesthesiologist to be alert for ventilatory compromise as indicated by increased peak airway pressures and decreased pulse oximetry. Young healthy patients with normal body mass indices generally do not have any clinically relevant alterations in respiration or ventilation.

Insufflation of CO_2 produces hemodynamic changes in CO, SVR, and venous return. These changes become pronounced and complicated to address when the patient is placed in various tilt positions. The head down position produces an increase in venous return, therefore an increase in central venous pressure (CVP) and a concomitant increase in CO. Healthy patients can tolerate this increased myocardial workload. However, patients with cardiovascular disease or those with ventricular dysfunction may not be able to withstand this change in myocardial oxygen demand, and myocardial insult may occur.

When positioning patients on the operating room table peripheral nerves become vulnerable to injury. The ulnar nerve is the most commonly injured nerve during surgery. Padding each elbow is necessary to help protect the nerve. The common peroneal nerve is susceptible to compression, especially in the lithotomy position. Stretching of the sciatic nerve and compression of the obturator, femoral, and lateral femoral cutaneous nerves also may occur with the hips and legs flexed in this position. The lateral decubitus position requires an axillary roll to be placed to prevent stretching of the brachial plexus.

2.4. Laparoscopic Robotic Surgery

The introduction of robotics to urologic surgery has expanded the benefits of laparoscopy and introduced specific anesthetic considerations. The anesthesiologist has a responsibility to ensure immobility, proper positioning of the patient and protecting the patient from inadvertent injury by the movable robotic arms. Once the robotic system is locked into position the patient must remain in a fixed position throughout the operation. Therefore, precise patient positioning is required at the beginning of the case. This obviates the need for complete muscle relaxation and prevents the augmentation of hemodynamics through changes in position. If the patient must be moved for any reason the robotic instruments must first be removed from the patient, and then the instruments are disassembled from the robotic arms and the robotic system is "undocked," allowing movement of the patient. The vigilant anesthesi-

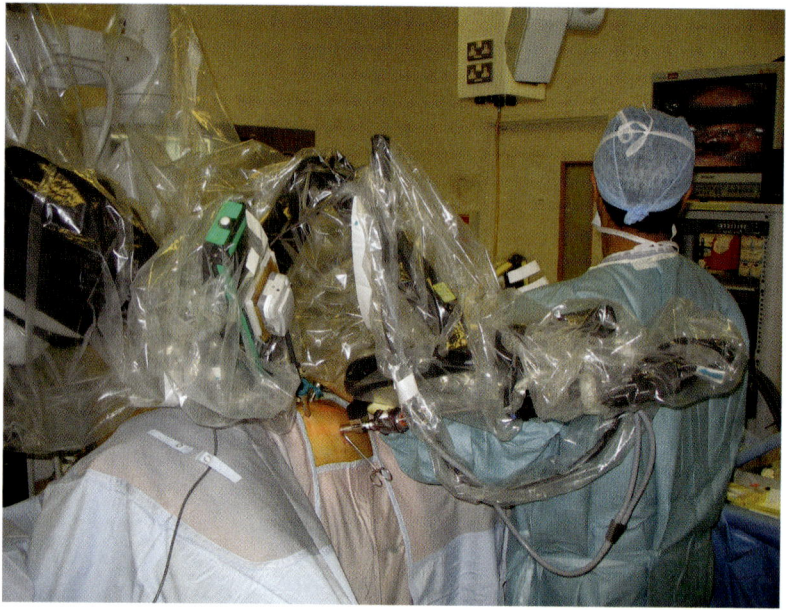

Fig. 1. Careful positioning and padding of the patient is mandatory to ensure protection of the patient from the movable robotic arms.

ologist also must ensure that the patient is protected from the moving robotic arms, which could lead to injury (Fig. 1).

3. PREOPERATIVE CONSIDERATIONS

3.1. Preoperative Evaluation

A directed anesthetic pre-operative evaluation consists of a detailed history and physical, discussion of previous anesthetic experiences and a detailed examination of the patients airway. The physiological changes and specialized positioning of the patient during laparoscopic surgeries require that the patient have adequate respiratory and cardiovascular reserve. Patient's deemed unfit to compensate for hemodynamic and pulmonary fluctuations may benefit from an open procedure. The anesthesiologist must pay particular attention to the respiratory and cardiovascular functional status. A focused inquiry into the patient's respiratory history is paramount. The physician must obtain information regarding; wheezing, recent respiratory tract infections, obstructive or restrictive disease, and a smoking history, all of which decrease pulmonary function and inhibit reserve capacity. Excess body weight and its' distribution also must be evaluated. Patients with large adipose deposits in the mid

Table 1
ASA classification system to determine relative risks of perioperative morbidity
and mortality

Status	Disease state	Mortality (%)
ASA Class 1	A normal healthy patient	0.06–0.08
ASA Class 2	A patient with mild systemic disease that results in no functional limitations, i.e., hypertension, diabetes, extremes of age	0.27–0.4
ASA Class 3	A patient with severe systemic disease that results in functional limitations, i.e., uncontrolled hypertension, angina, prior MI, pulmonary disease that limits activity	1.8–4.3
ASA Class 4	A patient with severe systemic disease that is a constant threat to life, i.e., CHF, unstable angina, advanced pulmonary, renal or hepatic dysfunction	7.8–23
ASA Class 5	A moribund patient who is not expected to survive without the operation, i.e., ruptured abdominal aneurysm, head injury with increased ICP	9.4–51
ASA Class 6	A declared brain dead patient whose organs are being removed for donor purposes	
Emergency (E)	Any patient in whom an emergency operation is required	

abdomen have increased ventilation perfusion mismatch, especially when supine because of the diaphragmatic compression on the base of the lungs. The cardiac evaluation should include a history of coronary artery disease, valvular disease and exercise tolerance. The patient's ability to climb two flights of stairs suggests a myocardium that can tolerate surgical stress (26). The ASA classification system stratifies patients into categories to determine the relative risks of perioperative morbidity and mortality (Table 1).

3.2. Laboratory Evaluation

Preoperative testing recommendations have been established by the ASA to serve as a guideline for the practitioner to optimize outcomes. A case specific approach with a tailored investigation is both cost-effective and beneficial to overall preoperative management. For example, a 25-year old male with no prior medical history does not require any preoperative laboratory testing. A 30-year-old female may only require a pregnancy test and baseline hemoglobin before surgery. However, patients with a significant medical history and those taking medications require directed laboratory evaluation. For example; patients taking diuretics require a basic metabolic panel to evaluate serum potassium levels and other electrolytes, diabetics require perioperative blood glucose levels, and patients with a significant cardiac history may require a full cardiac evaluation. These individual decisions are best made in consult with the anesthesiologist. Table 2 lists the recommendations for ASA class 1 patients.

3.3. Anesthetic Techniques

A variety of anesthetic techniques may be used during laparoscopic surgery. By understanding the advantages and disadvantages of each technique, the physician can optimize care. The duration of the surgery is a primary consideration when choosing the anesthetic plan. General anesthesia with endotracheal intubation is preferred in most cases. The advantages include definitive airway protection, the ability to provide deep muscle relaxation and positive pressure ventilation. The laryngeal mask airway also may be used, but it is generally not recommended. If peak airway pressures exceed 20 mmHg, the lower esophageal sphincter may be overcome, leading to gastric content regurgitation and an increased risk of aspiration. Regional anesthesia is another method that may be performed. However, patient cooperation is required during the specialized positions, in addition, a nasogastric or orogastric tube is often placed to decompress the stomach, which may not be tolerated as well in a conscious patient. General anesthesia is therefore the method of choice for most laparoscopic surgeries.

Table 2
Recommendations[a] for ASA class 1 patients

Age (healthy)	Male	Female
<40	No tests needed	If menstruating: B-hcg, H/H
40–64	ECG	If menstruating: B-hcg, H/H ECG
>64	ECG, CXR	ECG, CXR

[a]ECG, electrocardiogram; CXR, chest X-ray; B-hcg, β-human chorionic gonadotropin; H/H, Hemoglobin/Hematocrit

4. INTRAOPERATIVE CONSIDERATIONS AND RISKS OF LAPAROSCOPIC SURGERY

The complications of performing endoscopic surgery vary in severity. The prudent surgeon and anesthesiologist must consider all potential risks associated with minimally invasive procedures.

The introduction of the Veress needle or trocar may cause vascular damage. Vessels may be injured and bleed into the surgical field, or they may be concealed within the retroperitoneal space. Early signs of concealed bleeding are tachycardia, decreased urine output, and hypotension, which may be refractory to fluid boluses. Hemorrhage in this location must be considered if unexplained hypotension is noted. Immediate conversion to an open procedure is indicated to control and repair injured vessels.

Cardiac arrhythmias, such as bradycardia and asystole have been observed. This is due to either vagal stimulation during insufflation of gas or the increase in $PaCO_2$ *(26)*. All patients require standard cardiac monitoring during laparoscopic surgery. Patients with a known cardiac history should have five lead analyses intraoperatively.

Subcutaneous emphysema is yet another complication that may occur when the Veress needle tip is improperly placed into a cavity. Insufflated gas may dissect planes of tissue, exposing capillaries to CO_2, resulting in hypercapnia. Data from laparoscopic cholecystectomy suggest an incidence of subcutaneous emphysema as high as 0.4–2% *(26)*. The clinician can identify this complication by palpating crepitus over the affected site. No specific treatment is available for subcutaneous emphysema other than supportive care and pain management.

The physician must be able to recognize and treat the development of a pneumomediastinum or pneumothorax. Pneumomediastinum is generated when gas escapes the abdomen and travels into the thoracic cavity, at the level of T10, through the esophageal hiatus. Additionally, gas may enter the thorax via preexisting defects in the diaphragm. A pneumothorax is created when increased pressure on the external parietal pleura leads to pleura rupture *(26)*. Treatment depends on the extent of the pneumothorax and the clinical presentation. Patients with cardiovascular collapse require immediate needle decompression followed by chest tube insertion and discontinuing insufflation.

A venous gas CO_2 embolism is created when CO_2 lodges inside a blood vessel. There are different mechanisms by which a CO_2 embolism is generated; the inadvertent injection of CO_2 directly into a vein or gas being drawn into an open vessel. The size and location are critical in determining the severity of symptoms. A large gas emboli in any of the great vessels can be catastrophic for patients. Hypoxemia, hypotension, tachycardia, and a transient decrease in end tidal CO_2 support the diagnosis of a significant gas embolism. A transesophageal echocardiogram or precordial Doppler are both sensitive tests for the diagnosis of an embolism. Treatment includes discontinuation of CO_2 gas insufflation and placing the patient in the Trendelenburg position whenever possible. Ideally, a multiport central venous catheter should be placed, preferably in the right internal jugular vein, and the gas emboli should be aspirated from the right ventricle.

5. POSTOPERATIVE CONSIDERATIONS AND MANAGEMENT TECHNIQUES

5.1. Postoperative Nausea and Vomiting (PONV)

PONV is commonly referred to as "The big little problem in anesthesia." Much has been written about PONV due to its high incidence and its impact on the postoperative course. Up to 75% of patients may complain of nausea, vomiting, or both after laparoscopic surgery (27–29). PONV is the most common postoperative complication that leads directly to delayed discharge and or hospital admission (30,31). The cause of nausea is thought to be due to a sudden increase in intra-abdominal pressure from gas inflation. Stretching of the peritoneal fibers elicits afferent neurogenic pathways that activate the chemoreceptor trigger zone in the brainstem leading to nausea. A perioperative risk analysis and tailored pharmacologic approach are necessary for each patient to prevent this untoward effect. A risk stratification based on the following factors is used to identify who is at greatest risk. According to the consensus guidelines, there are four independent factors that contribute to PONV (32).

1. Female.
2. Nonsmoker.
3. History of PONV or motion sickness.
4. Use of opioids perioperatively.

Each independent factor is additive; therefore, two or more risk factors place the patient at a great risk for PONV. These risk factors are independent of the type of procedure being performed, even though certain surgeries such as laparoscopy, gynecological, plastics, and eye and ear are associated with a high incidence of PONV. Therefore, recommended prophylaxis is based exclusively on the four factors. An algorithm has been created to manage PONV (Fig. 2).

The guidelines also recommend a strategy for initial therapy of PONV and therapy for those who failed prophylaxis (Table 3).

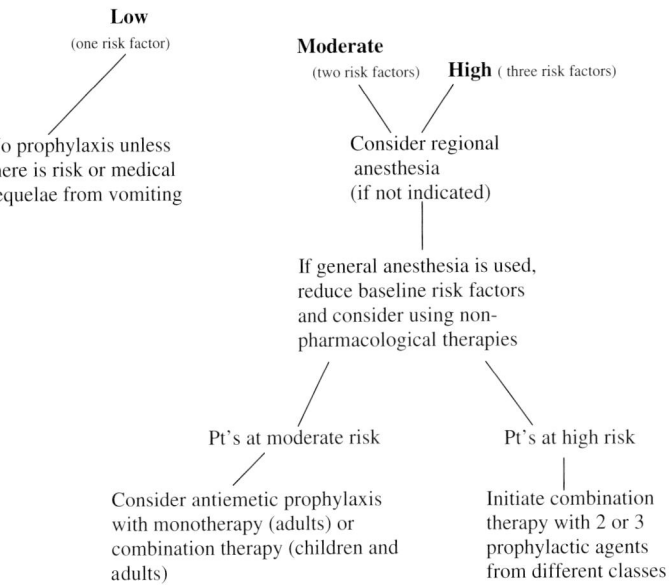

Fig. 2. Risk of PONV.

5.2. Pain Management

Laparoscopic procedures are known to cause less pain and discomfort than classic open procedures *(33–35)*. Although these procedures are considered "minimally invasive," the type and severity of pain seen postoperatively is both visceral and somatic, and it can be very intense. Visceral pain is due to organ distension after gas insufflation. Somatic pain is due to port site incisions and body wall distension. In addition, referred pain to the right shoulder is common as a result of diaphragmatic irritation from the insufflated gas *(36)*. Current recommendations for the management of postoperative pain include a multimodal approach that starts preoperatively. Preemptive nonsteroidal anti-inflammatory drugs (NSAIDs), opioids, or both may be given before the induction of anesthesia, and they may even be started the evening before surgery if instructed to do so after a preanesthetic evaluation. Preventative dosing has been shown to be very successful in treating surgical pain and is recommended for all cases. In addition, intraoperative local anesthetic injection of the port sites is an excellent way to inhibit somatic pain. Bupivacaine (0.25%) at a maximum dose of 2.5 mg/kg is a commonly

Table 3
Strategy for initial therapy of PONV and therapy for those who failed
prophylaxis

Initial therapy	Failed prophylaxis
No prophylaxis	Administer small dose 5-HT$_3$ antagonist [a]
Serotonin (5-HT$_3$) antagonist[a] plus second agent[b]	Use drug from different class. Do not repeat initial therapy
Triple therapy with 5-HT$_3$ antagonist[a] plus two other agents[b] when PONV occurs <6 h after surgery	Use drug from different class. Use drug from different class or propofol, 20 mg as needed in postanesthesia care unit
Triple therapy with 5-HT$_3$ antagonist[a] plus two other agents[b] when PONV occurs >6 h after surgery	Repeat 5-HT$_3$ antagonist[a] and droperidol (not dexamethasone or transdermal scopolamine)

[a]Small dose 5-HT$_3$ antagonist dosing: 1.0 mg of ondansetron, 12.5 mg of dolasetron, 0.1 mg of granisetron, and 0.5 mg of tropisetron.
[b]Alternative therapies for rescue: droperidol (0.625 mg i.v.), dexamethasone (2–4 mg i.v.), and promethazine (12.5 mg i.v.).
Reprinted with permission from Gan et al. (2003) Anesth Analg 97:62–71.

used local anesthetic for incision site infiltration. Postoperative NSAIDs may prove to be beneficial as well as i.v. opioids.

6. SUMMARY

The advent of laparoscopy has afforded many advances in urologic surgery. The introduction of robotic technology will further enhance what can be accomplished in the name of better patient care. Having a thorough treatment plan in consult with the anesthesiologist allows this technology to be most effectively implemented from the preoperative evaluation to intraoperative management and postoperative care.

REFERENCES

1. Clayman RV, Kavoussi LR (1992) Endosurgical techniques for the diagnosis and treatment of noncalculus disease of the ureter and kidney. In: Walsh P, Retik A, Stamey T et al (eds), Campbell's urology, 6th edn. W. B. Saunders, Philadelphia, PA, p 2231.
2. O'Hara JF Jr, Cywinski JB, Monk TG (2006) The renal system and anesthesia for urologic surgery. In: Barash PG, Cullen BF, Stoelting RK (eds) Clinical anesthesia, 5th edn. Lippincott Williams & Wilkins, Philadelphia, PA, pp 1013–1035.

3. Mullett CE, Viale JP, Sagnard PE et al (1993) Pulmonary CO_2 elimination during surgical procedures using intra- or extraperitoneal CO_2 insufflation. Anesth Analg 76:622.

4. Joris JL (2005) Anesthesia for laparoscopic surgery. In: Miller RD (ed) Miller's anesthesia, 6th edn. Elsevier Churchill Livingstone, Philadelphia, PA, pp 2285–2306.

5. Joris JL, Noirot DP, Legrand MJ et al (1993) Hemodynamic changes during laparoscopic cholecystectomy. Anesth Analg 76:1067.

6. Joris JL, Chiche JD, Canivet JL et al (1998) Hemodynamic changes induced by laparoscopy and their endocrine correlates: effects of clonidine. J Am Coll Cardiol 32:1389.

7. Odeberg S, Ljungqvist O, Svenberg T et al (1994) Hemodynamic effects of pneumoperitoneum and the influence of posture during anesthesia for laparoscopic surgery. Acta Anesthesiol Scand 38:276.

8. Safran DB, Orlando R 3rd (1994) Physiologic effects of pneumoperitoneum. Am J Surg 167:281.

9. Koivusalo AM, Lindgren L (2000) Effects of carbon dioxide pneumoperitoneum for laparoscopic cholecystectomy. Acta Anesthesiol Scand 44:834.

10. Ivankovich AD, Miletich DJ, Albrecath RF et al (1975) Cardiovascular effects of intraperitoneal insufflation with carbon dioxide insufflation and nitrous oxide in the dog. Anesthesiology 42:281.

11. Dexter SP, Vucevic M, Gibson J et al (1999) Hemodynamic consequences of high- and low- pressure capnoperitoneum during laparoscopic cholecystectomy. Surg Endosc 13:376.

12. Dorsay DA, Green FL, Baysinger CL (1995) Hemodynamic changes during laparoscopic cholecystectomy monitored with transesophageal echocardiography. Surg Endosc 9:128.

13. Ho HS, Saunders CJ, Corso FA et al (1993) The effects of CO_2 pneumoperitoneum on hemodynamics in hemorrhaged animals. Surgery 114:381.

14. Kashtan J, Green JF, Parsons EQ et al (1981) Hemodynamic effects of increased abdominal pressure. J Surg Res 30:249.

15. Alishahi S, Francis N, Crofts S et al (2001) Central and peripheral adverse hemodynamic changes during laparoscopic surgery and their reversal with a novel intermittent sequential pneumatic compression device. Ann Surg 233:176.

16. Hirvonen EA, Nuutinen LS, Vuolteenaho O (1997) Hormonal responses and cardiac filling pressures in head up or head down position and pneumoperitoneum in patients undergoing operative laparoscopy. Br J Anaesth 78:128.

17. O'Leary E, Hubbard K, Tormey W et al (1996) Laparoscopic cholecystectomy: hemodynamic and neuroendocrine responses after pneumoperitoneum and changes in position. Br J Anasth 76:640.

18. Mann C, Boccara G, Pouzeratte Y et al (1999) The relationship among carbon dioxide pneumoperitoneum, vasopressin release, and hemodynamic changes. Anesth Analg 89:279.

19. Pepine CJ, Lambert CR (1990) Cardiovascular effects of nicardipine. Angiology 41:978.

20. Brantley JC 3rd, Riley PM (1988) Cardiovascular collapse during laparoscopy: a report of two cases. Am J Obstet Gynecol 159:735.

21. Weingram J (2003) Laparoscopic surgery. In: Yao FF (ed) Anesthesiology problem-oriented patient management, 5th edn. Lippincott Williams & Wilkins, Philadelphia, PA, pp 858–888.

22. Cunningham AJ, Turner J, Rosenbaum S et al (1993) Transesophageal assessment of hemodynamic function during laparoscopic cholecystectomy. Br J Anaesth 70:621.

23. Rasmussen JP, Dauchot PJ, De Palma RG (1978) Cardiac function and hypercarbia. Arch Surg 113:1196.

24. Wolf JS Jr, Carrier S, Stoller ML (1994) Gas embolism: helium is more lethal than carbon dioxide. J Laparoendosc Surg 4:173.

25. Roberts MW, Mathiesen KA, Ho HS et al (1997) Cardiopulmonary responses to intervenous infusion of soluble and relatively insoluble gases. Surg Endosc 11:341.

26. Cunningham AJ, Nolan C (2006) Anesthesia for minimally invasive procedures. In: Barash PG, Cullen BF, Stoelting RK (eds) Clinical anesthesia, 5th edn. Lippincott Williams & Wilkins, Philadelphia, PA, pp 1061–1071.

27. Bailey PL, Streisand JB, Pace NL et al (1990) Transdermal scopolamine reduces nausea and vomiting after outpatient laparoscopy. Anesthesiology 72:977.

28. Watcha MF, White PF (1992) Postoperative nausea and vomiting. Its' etiology, treatment, and prevention. Anesthesiology 77:162.

29. Beattie WS, Lindblad T, Buckley DN et al (1993) Menstruation increases the risk of nausea and vomiting after laparoscopy. A randomized study. Anesthesiology 78:272.

30. Gold BS, Kitz DS, Lecky JH, Neuhaus JM (1989) Unanticipated admission to the hospital following ambulatory surgery. J Am Med Assoc 262:3008–3010.

31. Fortier J, Chung F, Su J (1998) Unanticipated admission after ambulatory surgery: a prospective study. Can J Anaesth 45:612–619.

32. Gan Tong J et al (2003) Consensus guidelines for managing postoperative nausea and vomiting. Anesth Analg 97:62–71.

33. Joris J, Cigarini I, Legrand M et al (1992) Metabolic and respiratory changes after cholecystectomy performed via laparotomy or laparoscopy. Br J Anaesth 69:341.

34. Mealy K, Gallagher H, Barry M et al (1992) Physiological and metabolic responses to open and laparoscopic cholecystectomy. Br J Surg 79:1061.

35. Rademaker BM, Ringers J, Odoom JA et al (1992) Pulmonary function and stress response after laparoscopic cholecystectomy: comparison with subcostal incision and influence of thoracic epidural analgesia. Anesth Analg 75:381.

36. Joris J, Thiry E, Paris P et al (1995) Pain after laparoscopic cholecystectomy: characteristics and effect of intraperitoneal bupivacaine. Anesth Analg 81:379.

Index

A

Abdominal surgeries, prior, 108
AESOP, *see* Automated
    Endoscopic System
    for Optimal Positioning
    (AESOP)
Allen stirrups, 50
American Society of
    Anesthesiology (ASA), 216
  class-one patients,
    recommendations, 222
  perioperative
    morbidity/mortality risks,
    classification system, 221
Antibiotic prophylaxis, 73, 112, 145
Arterial bleeding, minor/major,
    see Hemostasis
ASA, *see* American Society of
    Anesthesiology (ASA)
Asimov, Isaac, 14
Automated Endoscopic System for
    Optimal Positioning
    (AESOP), 23, 24, 179
Automaton, 3, 4, 6, 9

B

Balloon dissection, 44
  See also Extraperitoneal/
    retroperitoneal
    laparoscopy
Brown, Dan, 6

C

Capek, Karel, 11
Carter-Thomason device, 44, 186

Central venous pressure
    (CVP), 219
Clepsydra (water clock), 4
CO_2 absorption/accumulation,
    laparoscopic surgery,
    217–218
Cobra, fourth robotic arm, *see*
    Pro-Grasp, the fourth arm
Computed tomography (CT)
    angiography, 128
Credentialing, robotic-assisted
    surgery, 212
Credentialing requirements,
    robot-assisted surgery,
    209–211
  attending physicians, 211
  monitoring, 211
  nonphysicians/physician,
    209–210
  recommendations, 211
CVP, *see* Central venous pressure
    (CVP)
Cystoprostatectomy, 89, 90
Cystourethroscopy, 148, 149

D

da Vinci, Leonardo, *see*
    Renaissance man
"The da Vinci Code," 6
da Vinci Surgical System, 20–24
  components, 148–149
    control tower, 131
    surgeon console, 130
    surgical arm cart, 131
DeBakey forceps, 140, 142, 149, 152

Denans' rings, 172
Detrusorrhaphy, 152
Donor nephrectomy (robotic),
    125–136
  complications, management
      of, 136
    intraoperative,
        vascular/ureter, 136
  instrumentation
    laparoscopic, 130
    robotic, 128–129
  kidney donation
    nonliving/living related
        donors, 125
    preoperative evaluation,
        donor, 129
  operating room setup, robotic
      system, 130–132
  postoperative care, 135–136
  preoperative assessment, 128
  surgical anatomy, 127–128
  surgical technique
    anterior dissection
        of kidney, 134
    colon mobilization and ureter
        identification, 133–134
    dissection of renal hilum, 135
    hook electrocautery, 133
    kidney, posterior dissection
        of, 134
    patient position, 132
    port placement, 132–133
    postoperative
        performance, 136
    renal hilum and kidney
        removal, division of, 135
Duodenum, Kocherized, 116

E

Elective hemostasis
  nephrectomy, partial, 191–195
    cigar method, 194
    FloSeal, 195
    Harmonic Scalpel, 192
      percutaneous radiofrequency
          coagulation, renal
          tumors, 194
      surgical adhesives,
          comparison of (table), 196
      Tisseel VH, 195
      venting the abdomen, argon
          beam coagulator, 193
  prostatectomy, radical,
      195–197
    dorsal vein, handling, 197
    LigaSure, use of, 197
    See also Hemostasis
Ergonomics, robotic suturing,
    173–174
Ethicon extra-long articulating
    laparoscopic stapler (ETS
    Flex 45), 92
Ethicon purple Hasson port, 186
Extraperitoneal/retroperitoneal
    laparoscopy, 43–44
  balloon dissection,
      extraperitoneal space, 44

F

Female cystectomy, 108
FloSeal, 99, 105, 115,
    119, 195
Flute Player, 6
Foley catheter, 39, 55, 75, 79, 82,
    119, 122, 132, 136, 140, 142,
    144, 149, 189, 201
Food and Drug Administration
    (FDA), 18, 19, 22, 24, 208
Fowler-Stephens technique, 166
The Franklin Institute Science
    museum in Philadelphia, 9

G

Gibson (lower)/Pfannenstiel
    incision, 118
"Gold standard," open
    dismembered
    pyeloplasty, 139

H

Haptic feedback, 19, 64, 176,
    177, 178
Harmonic Scalpel, 188, 191, 192
Hasson technique, 42, 52, 108, 142,
    144, 149, 151, 163, 187, 202
  advantages, 42–43
  incision procedure, purposes, 42
Hemostasis, 105, 185–197
  avoidance, 186–188
    electrocautery,
      mono/bipolar, 187
    Ethicon purple Hasson
      port, 186
    Hasson technique, use of, 187
    LigaSure Vessel Sealing
      System, 188
    preperitoneal approach,
      pelvic surgery, 187
  blood stain on tissues,
    effects, 185
  elective, see Elective hemostasis
  major arterial bleeding, 190–191
  major venous bleeding, 189–190
    Yasergil vascular clamps,
      189–190
  minor arterial bleeding, 190–191
  minor venous bleeding, 188–189
    suction cannula, 188
  preparation, 185–186
HLA, see Human lymphocyte
    antigens (HLA)
Human lymphocyte antigens
    (HLA), 128

I

IAT, see Intra-abdominal testis
    (IAT)
IAVT, see Intra-abdominal
    "vanishing" testis (IAVT)
Intra-abdominal testis (IAT), 159
Intra-abdominal "vanishing" testis
    (IAVT), 160
Intracorporeal suturing, 160, 174

Intravenous fluid replacement
    (IVF), 73
IVF, see Intravenous fluid
    replacement (IVF)

K

Kidney donor preoperative
    evaluation, 129
Kidney morcellation, 118
Kocher mobilization,
    duodenum, 116

L

Laparoscopic LigaSure Vessel
    Sealing System, 188
Laparoscopic radical
    prostatectomy (LRP), 49,
    61, 62, 63, 64, 66, 71, 72
Laparoscopy(ic)
  extraperitoneal/retroperitoneal,
    43–44
  intraoperative considerations
    and risks of, 223–224
  robotic surgery, 219–220
  suturing and knot-tying, 179
Last supper period, 6
Laws of robotics (Asimov's), 11
Lich–Gregoir technique, 147
LigaSure, 130, 135, 186, 188, 197
LRP, see Laparoscopic radical
    prostatectomy (LRP)

M

Maillardet, Henri, 9
Medical Forward Area Surgical
    Team (MEDFAST), 19
Mobile Advance Surgical Hospital
    (MASH), 19
Murphy button, 173

N

NASA (National Aeronautics and
    Space Administration),
    13, 18

Nasogastric/orogastric tube
        decompression, 92, 100,
        102, 121, 163, 201, 222
Neobladder-urethral
        anastomosis, 91
Nephrectomy, partial elective
        hemostasis, *see* Elective
        hemostasis
Nephrectomy/partial
        nephrectomy/
        nephroureterectomy,
        robotic laparoscopy,
        111–123
    complications, 121–123
    instruments, 113–115
    nephrectomy procedure,
        116–118
        Kocher mobilization,
            duodenum, 116
        Weck Hem-o-Lok polymer
            clip, 117
    nephroureterectomy bladder
        cuff procedure, 120–121
    operating room configuration
        and patient positioning,
        112–113
    partial nephrectomy procedure,
        118–119
        open collecting system
            defects, 119
    postoperative management, 121
        nasogastric/orogastric tube
            decompression, 121
    preoperative preparation, 112
    specimen removal, 118
        Gibson (lower)/Pfannenstiel
            incision, 118
        kidney morcellation, 118
    trocar placement, 115–116
Neurovascular bundles (NVB), 56,
        61, 80–82, 96–99
NVB, *see* Neurovascular bundles
        (NVB)

O
Operating room setup,
        patient/instrument
        preparation
    aparoscopic baskets, creation,
        29–30
    case, set up, 32–33
        robotic video cart,
            positioning, 33
        video cart, positioning, 33
    positioning, patient, 33–36
    robotic equipment,
        organizing/creating/
        handling, 30–32
        accessory basket, creation, 30
        ultrasonic cleaning, 31
        upkeep, 31
    surgeon preference card,
        creation, 32
        items, basic, 32
        trocar, disposable, 32
Orchiopexy (robotic)
    complications, management
        of, 168
    instrumentation, 162–163
    laparoscopic view
        of IAT, 162
        of normal right internal
            inguinal ring (figure), 161
    literature review, 160
        PubMed, 160
    operating room setup, 163
    patient position, 163
    port placement, 163–164
        for a right IAT (figure), 164
    port positioning for a bilateral
        IAT (figure), 165
    preoperative assessment,
        161–162
    special considerations, 168
    step-by-step approach,
        165–167
        Fowler–Stephens
            technique, 166

IAVT, diagnosis of, 165
intrauterine torsion,
    descended testes, 165
surgical procedures, 166
surgical anatomy, 160–161

P

Pain management, laparoscopic
    procedure, 225
Parker–Kerr running closure, 100
Patient/instrument preparation,
    see Operating room setup,
    patient/instrument
    preparation
Patient positioning, laparoscopic
    surgery, 218–219
Plasma-kinetic (PK) dissector, 53,
    55, 56, 59
Pneumoperitoneum, 41, 44, 45, 78,
    91, 99, 102, 105, 109, 112,
    122, 132, 142, 164, 195, 203,
    216–218
    dysrhythmias, 217
    hemodynamics, 216–217
PONV, *see* Postoperative nausea
    and vomiting (PONV)
Port placement and exit, 39–45
    complications, 45
        bowel/trocar/vascular
            injury, 45
    extraperitoneal/retroperitoneal
        laparoscopy, 43–44
    Hasson technique (open), 42–43
    secondary port placement, 43
        internal/external
            monitoring, 43
    trocar removal and port
        closure, 44–45
        Carter-Thomason closure
            device, 45
    veress needle access, *see* Veress
        needle access (closed
        technique)

Postoperative nausea and
    vomiting (PONV),
    224–225, 226
    risk of, 225
    therapy, initial
        strategy/prophylaxis
        failure, 226
Preperitoneal approach,
    advantages, 52
PROBOT surgical robotic system
    (figure), 18
Programmable Universal Machine
    for Assembly (PUMA), 12,
    15, 17
Pro-Grasp, the fourth arm, 94, 96,
    99, 102, 103, 105
Prostate cancer, oncologic cure,
    63–66
Prostatectomy, extraperitoneal
    robotic radical
    anesthetic considerations, 73–74
    bladder neck, localization and
        opening of, 78–79
    dorsal venous complex and
        urethra, transection, 81–82
    endopelvic fascia opening,
        78–79
    extraperitoneal access, 75
    neurovascular bundle
        dissection/sparing, 81
    patient positioning, 74–75
    pelvic space cleaning, 78
    posterior bladder neck
        transection, 79–80
    preoperative assessment, 72–73
        flexible cystoscopy, 73
    running anastomosis, 82–83
        TRUS biopsy, 82
    salvage of extraperitoneal
        space, 76
    seminal vesicle and vasa
        dissection, 80–81
    trocar insertion, 75–76

trocars/robotic arms to
  continue extraperitoneal
  procedure, positioning of,
  77–78
undocking, 83
Prostatectomy, transperitoneal
  (robotic)
anterior bladder neck
  dissection, 55
apical dissection, 56
denonvilliers' fascia and
  posterior dissection, 56
endopelvic fascia and ligation
  of dorsal venous complex,
  incision of, 53
lymph node dissection, 56, 59
peritoneum and entry into
  retropubic space, incision
  of, 53
posterior bladder neck, 55
retrograde (early) athermal
  preservation, NVB, 56
seminal vesicle dissection,
  55–56
urethrovesical anastomosis, 59
Pyeloplasty (robotic), 139–144
complications, management of
  intraoper-
    ative/postoperative, 144
instrumentation, 140
patient position and port
  placement, 140
preoperative assessment,
  139–140
special considerations, 143
  antegrade stent
    placement, 143
step-by-step approach, 140–143
  additional ports, 142
  Betadine skin prep, 142
  layers of dissection,
    identification, 142
  ports, children, 142

R
Radical cystectomy, robotic
  laparoscopy, 89–109
complications, management
  of, 109
considerations
  arm or pubic bone
    interference, 107
  collisions and robotic
    operating
    reach/range, 106
  external elbow SUJ
    adjustments, 107
  female cystectomy, 108
  fourth arm, 105–106
  hemostasis, 105
  obese patients, 108
  orthotopic neobladder
    mesenteric length, 105
  port remote center
    adjustments, 106
  port sites and urinary
    diversion, 106
  prior abdominal
    surgeries, 108
  respiratory conditions, 109
  specimen removal, 104–105
  urethral anastomosis, 105
  urethrectomy, 108–109
instrumentation and operating
  room setup, 92
port placements, 94
postoperative management, 104
preoperative assessment, 91–92
  stoma
    counseling/marking, 92
surgical anatomy
  considerations, 90–91
surgical technique, see Robotic
  surgical technique
Radical prostatectomy, 195–197
See also Elective hemostasis
Radical retropublic prostatectomy
  (RRP), 49, 50, 61–64

Radionuclide cystogram
    (RNC), 148
RALP, *see* Robotic transperitoneal
    four arm laparoscopic
    radical prostatectomy
    (RALP)
Renaissance man, 4
    See also da Vinci, Leonardo
Renal transplantation, 125
Retrograde/antegrade
    endopyelotomy, 139
rLRP, *see* Robotically assisted
    laparoscopic radical
    prostatectomy (rLRP)
RNC, *see* Radionuclide cystogram
    (RNC)
Robot
    coinage, 11
    definition/synonyms, 3
Robot-assisted surgery in urology
    competence, surgical, 211–212
    concept, 208
    credentialing, 208–211
        monitoring, 211
        nonphysician/physician,
            209–210
        recommendations, 211
        surgical assistant, 211
        See also Credentialing
            requirements,
            robot-assisted surgery
    master/slave relationship,
        technology, 208
Robotically assisted laparoscopic
    radical prostatectomy
    (rLRP), 71, 72
Robotic end wrist technology, 177
Robotic surgery, complications
    of patient selection, 199–200
        with extremely muscular
            abdominal walls, 200
        obese patients, 200
    pelvic procedures, 201–202
    pneumoperitoneum, 203–204

preoperative preparation,
    200–201
procedures, 201–204
    bleeding, 203
    Hasson technique, 202
    induction of anesthesia, 201
proper trocar placement, 202
rectal injuries, 202–203
renal procedures, 201
short laparoscopic procedures
    (cholecystectomy/hernia
    repair), 202
Robotic surgical technique
bladder neck, securing, 101
division of left bladder
    pedicles, 96
exposure and posterior
    dissection, 94–95
    Denonvilliers space, 94–95
    EndoShears dissection, 95
extracorporeal urinary
    diversion, 100
    gastrointestinal (GI)
        continuity,
        reestablishment, 100
    Parker–Kerr running
        closure, 100
history of, 1–25
left ureter/pelvic lymph node
    dissection, 95–96
    monopolar/bipolar
        electrocautery, 95
    Pro-Grasp, the fourth arm, 96
modifications, 72
prostate dissection, 98
prostate neurovascular bundle
    preservation, 98–99
    FloSeal/Tisseel hemostatic
        agents, 98
    Weck polymer Hem-o-Lok
        clips, 98
releasing bladder anteriorly,
    97–98

right ureter and pelvic lymph nodes, 97

ureteral reimplantation, 101–102
    red Robinson silk suture, 101–102

ureters, securing, 99–100

urethro-vesical anastomosis, 102–103

Robotic team, for robot-assisted surgery, 211

Robotic transperitoneal four arm laparoscopic radical prostatectomy (RALP), 49–66

functional outcomes
    continence, maintenance/return, 62–63
    erectile function, 61–62
    oncologic, 63–66

haptic feedback, lack of, 64

indications/contraindications, 50

outcomes, 59–61
    blood loss and transfusion, 59–61
    operative time, 59

technique, 50–59
    intra-abdominal access/trocar placement, 50–52
    operating room setup, 50
    patient positioning, 50
    transperitoneal robotic prostatectomy, 53–59

RRP, see Radical retropublic prostatectomy (RRP)

S

Secondary port, placement, 43

Setup joint (SUJ), 106, 107

Storz fascial closure device, 186

SUJ, see Setup joint (SUJ)

Surgical adhesives, comparison of (table), 196

Surgical staplers, 173

Surgical system, da Vinci, 20–24

Suturing, robotic
    cognitive benefits, 174–175
    3D visualization, surgical suturing, 175–176
    ergonomics, 173–174
        laparoscopic suturing, 173
    future application, 180–181
        nitinol U-clips for mitral valve repairs, 180–181
    hand and wrist problems, 173
    haptic feedback, 177
        robotic end wrist technology, application, 177
    intracorporeal, 174
    learning curves, 179–180
        ex vivo studies, 180
    methodology, 171–172
        systems approach/component evaluation, 171–172
    microsurgical anastomoses and tremor filtration
        vasovasotomy, 178
        Zeus robot, 178
    suture manipulation and narrow working view, 176–177
    modified suture, concept of, 177
    suture material, working with, 176–177
    theory/history, 172–173
        Denans' rings, 172
        "do no harm," 172
        inflammatory reaction, wound, 172
        Murphy button, 173
        surgical staplers, 173

SVR, *see* Systemic vascular
  resistance (SVR)
Systemic vascular resistance
  (SVR), 216–217, 219

T

Telesurgery, 19
Tesla, Nikola, 9
Tisseel, 99, 105, 119, 195
Trocar desig-
  nation/types/insertion
  technique, 41

U

UPJ, *see* Ureteropelvic junction
  (UPJ)
Ureteral reflux surgery (robotic)
  complications, management
    of, 153
  hemostasis, 153
  instrumentation, 148–149
  literature review, 146–147
    Politano–Leadbetter
      ureteroneocystostomy, 146
  operating room setup, 149
  patient position, 149
  port placement, 149–151
    operating room setup
      (figure), 150
    sites for (figure), 150
  preoperative assessment, 148
    cystourethroscopy, role
      of, 148
    VCUG, 148
  step-by-step approach, 151–153
  surgical anatomy
    pelvis, 148
Ureteropelvic junction (UPJ), 142
Urethral anastomosis, 105
Urethrectomy, 108–109
Urology, anesthetic considerations
  (laparoscopic procedures)
  history of laparoscopy, 215
  indications, 215

intraoperative considerations
  and risks, 223–224
  cardiac arrhythmias, 223
  pneumomediastinum, 223
  subcutaneous
    emphysema, 223
issues, 215–216
physiological effects
  of, 216–220
  CO_2 absorption and
    accumulation, 217–218
  laparoscopic robotic surgery,
    219–220
  patient positioning,
    219–220
  pneumoperitoneum,
    216–217
postoperative considera-
  tions/management
  techniques, 224–226
  pain management, 225–226
  postoperative nausea and
    vomiting (PONV),
    224–225
preoperative evaluation,
  220–222
  anesthetic techniques, 222
  laboratory evaluation,
    221–222

V

Vasovasotomy, 178
VCUG, *see* Voiding
  cystourethrogram (VCUG)
Venous bleeding, major/minor, *see*
  Hemostasis
Veress needle access (closed
  technique)
  confirmation tests, 40
  needle, usage, 40
  trendelenburg position, 40
  trocar desig-
    nation/types/insertion
    technique, 41

Vesicoureteral reflux (VUR), 145

Voiding cystourethrogram
          (VCUG), 148

VUR, *see* Vesicoureteral reflux
          (VUR)

VUR, endoscopic management
          of, 146

W

Walsh's anatomic radical
          prostatectomy, 72
Weck Hem-o-Lok polymer
          clip, 117

Y

Yasergil vascular clamps, 189–190

Printed in the United States of America